Dedication

To my beloved family, friends, colleagues, and clients—this book is the culmination of a lifetime of passion, study, and a deep calling to help others. It has been a journey pursued quietly, often unknown even to those closest to me, but driven always by an unwavering commitment to understanding the power of Cellular Vitality. Years ago, I realized that true health starts at the cellular level, and it has been my mission ever since to learn, teach, and heal through this fundamental truth.

To my family, thank you for being my strength. I hope these pages bring you closer to the heart of what has guided me for so many years. Your love has given me courage and kept me grounded in this journey.

To my friends and colleagues, I am grateful for your constant encouragement and curiosity. You have cheered every step forward, listened through every challenge, and been by my side every step of the way, motivating me to press forward. Your presence in my life has been a gift.

And to my clients, who have trusted me not only with your health but also with your hopes, thank you for walking this path with me. Your trust is my greatest honor and motivation, an incredible privilege I hold close to my heart. This book is a testament to the dedication we share in the pursuit of true health. I promise to continue learning, growing, and fighting for us.

Finally, to my faith—for the wake-up call in 1998 that redirected my life's work, allowing me to apply years of research through the lens of biblical teachings. That moment changed everything, setting me on a path to promote the body's amazing self-healing abilities, as God intended. Helping people heal and thrive has become my purpose, and I embrace this calling wholeheartedly. I am grateful for the strength and guidance that have carried me on this path.

"I can do all things through Christ who strengthens me."—Philippians 4:13
"For I will restore health to you, and your wounds I will heal,
declares the Lord." —Jeremiah 30:17
Thank you to each of you for being part of this journey. May Cellular Vitality inspire, guide, and support you toward a life of vibrant health.

With all my love,
Kelly

Cellular Vitality

Natural Strategies to Boost Self-Healing and Optimize Mitochondrial Health

By

Dr. Kelly Brink

Legal & Disclaimer

The information contained in this book and its contents is not designed to replace or take the place of any form of medical or professional advice; and is not meant to replace the need for independent medical, financial, legal or other professional advice or services, as may be required. The content and information in this book has been provided for educational and entertainment purposes only.

The content and information contained in this book has been compiled from sources deemed reliable, and it is accurate to the best of the Author's knowledge, information and belief. However, the Author cannot guarantee its accuracy and validity and cannot be held liable for any errors and/or omissions. Further, changes are periodically made to this book as and when needed. Where appropriate and/or necessary, you must consult a professional (including but not limited to your doctor, attorney, financial advisor or such other professional advisor) before using any of the suggested remedies, techniques, or information in this book.

Upon using the contents and information contained in this book, you agree to hold harmless the Author from and against any damages, costs, and expenses, including any legal fees potentially resulting from the application of any of the information provided by this book. This disclaimer applies to any loss, damages or injury caused by the use and application, whether directly or indirectly, of any advice or information presented, whether for breach of contract, tort, negligence, personal injury, criminal intent, or under any other cause of action.

You agree to accept all risks of using the information presented inside this book. You agree that by continuing to read this book, where appropriate and/or necessary, you shall consult a professional (including but not limited to your doctor, attorney, or financial advisor or such other advisor as needed) before using any of the suggested remedies, techniques, or information in this book.

Table of Contents

Introduction

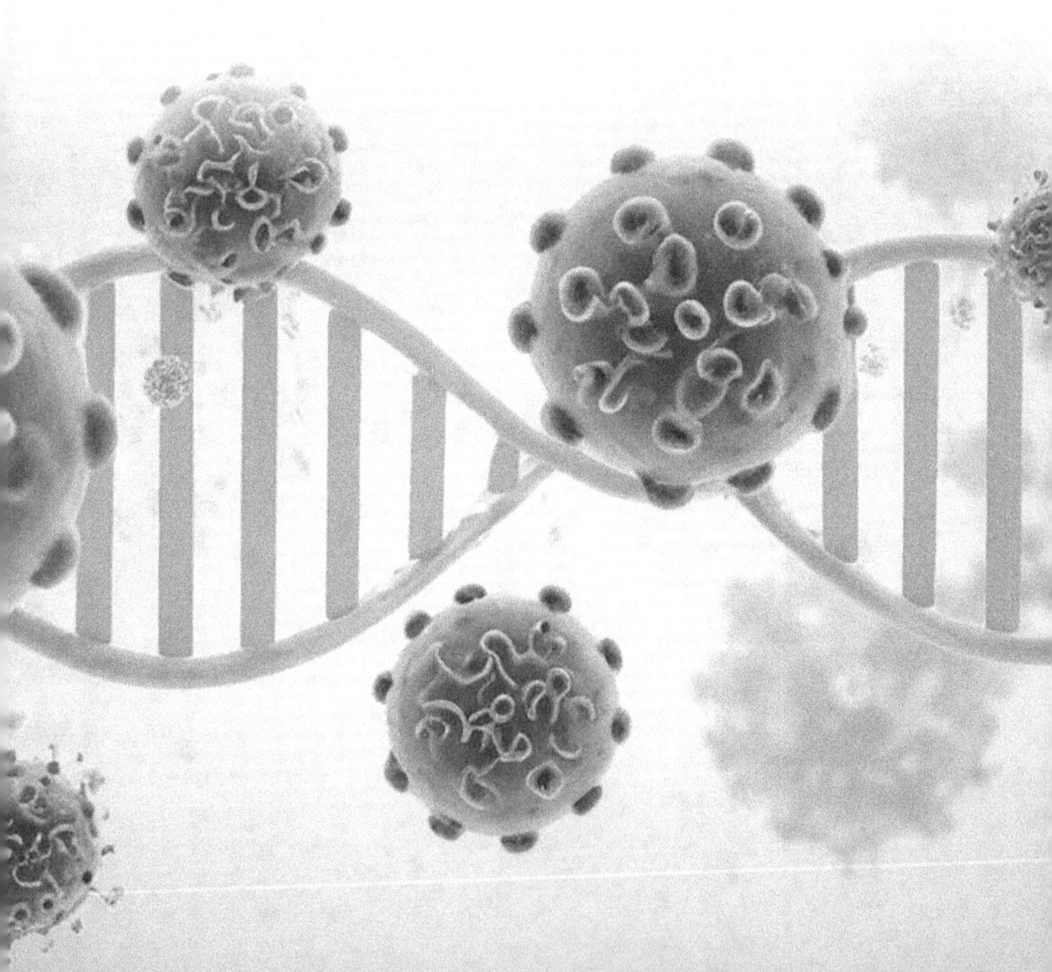

The phrase "Fix the cell to get and stay well" captures the essence of cellular health and serves as a reminder that by prioritizing the health of our cells—the very foundation of life—we can significantly improve our overall well-being. Healthy cells are essential for healing and longevity; when they function properly, they empower the body to recover and regenerate efficiently. Cellular health is at the core of understanding how the human body maintains itself, adapts to challenges, and ultimately thrives.

The body is composed of trillions of cells, each highly specialized to perform various functions essential for health and vitality. At the heart of every cell lies a nucleus containing DNA, the blueprint of life. Within this intricate framework are mitochondria—the "powerhouses" of the cell—that generate the energy required for cellular functions in the form of ATP (adenosine triphosphate). This energy production process is vital. A decline in cellular energy, mitochondrial dysfunction, or damage to cell membranes can lead to a wide range of health issues, from chronic fatigue and metabolic syndrome to neurodegenerative diseases and autoimmune disorders.

In 1998, I faced a health challenge that Western medicine could not resolve. It was during this time that I was officially labeled as a "sick person." Rather than accepting this fate, I returned to the research on mitochondrial function I had begun in 1993 and combined it with principles from biblical medicine. This journey—focused on targeting cellular health and optimizing the body's innate self-healing abilities—gave me my life back. Since then, it has been my mission to share this knowledge and approach to healing. This book is a passion project, one I've wanted to write since those early days.

By empowering our cells to heal, we give ourselves the best chance at living vibrant, fulfilling lives.

The Impact of Modern-Day Stressors on Cellular Health

Our bodies were intricately designed to function in a state of balance, known as homeostasis, where every system works harmoniously to maintain optimal health. This balance is fundamental to life itself. When we are in homeostasis, the body can adapt to changes, repair itself, and manage stress. However, the modern world presents a range of stressors that can disrupt this delicate equilibrium, throwing off our body's natural balance and leading to dysfunction at the cellular level. Poor diet, lack of sleep, environmental toxins, chronic emotional stress, and sedentary lifestyles all contribute to this imbalance. These stressors compound over time, tipping the scales toward disease rather than health.

Two major disruptors of cellular health in the modern world are insulin resistance and chronic inflammation. Insulin resistance occurs when cells in the muscles, fat, and liver begin to ignore the signal from insulin to absorb glucose from the blood. Over time, this can lead to elevated blood sugar levels and may result in Type 2 diabetes, weight gain, cardiovascular disease, and more. Chronic inflammation, on the other hand, is the body's sustained response to stressors or perceived threats. While inflammation is a natural and beneficial response to injury or infection, prolonged or "silent" inflammation at the cellular level can damage tissues. It is now recognized as a common underlying factor in many chronic diseases, including heart disease, cancer, and Alzheimer's disease.

Together, insulin resistance and chronic inflammation form a vicious cycle that not only fuels cellular damage but also disrupts the body's natural ability to repair itself. These conditions are insidious, often progressing silently without obvious symptoms until significant damage has occurred. The cumulative effect is a body that becomes increasingly inefficient at self-repair, energy production, and detoxification.

Why Cellular Health Matters

When we view the human body through the lens of cellular health, it becomes clear that every process, function, and system depends on the well-being of our cells. Whether it's the brain sending signals through neurons, the immune system fighting an infection, or the heart pumping blood, every action depends on healthy, well-functioning cells. Focusing on cellular health allows us to address health at its most fundamental level, creating a stable, resilient foundation upon which all other aspects of health can be built.

The science of cellular health is rich with potential. Recent studies have shown that we can influence our cellular function through specific lifestyle changes. For example, a study published in the Journal of Cell Biology highlights how optimizing cellular energy through mitochondrial support can increase resilience to stress, improve cognitive function, and even slow the aging process. Mitochondria are not only crucial for energy production but also for regulating the health of the cell, and by extension, the health of the body as a whole.

The Importance of a Holistic Approach to Wellness

A central theme throughout this book is the need for a holistic approach to wellness. It can be tempting to think that we can "fix" cellular health by focusing on just one aspect, such as diet or exercise. However, cellular health is an interconnected process, with each area of wellness—nutrition, sleep, stress management, movement, and mindfulness—playing a crucial role.

Nutrition provides the essential building blocks for cellular repair, regeneration, and protection against oxidative stress. A nutrient-dense, anti-inflammatory diet, rich in whole foods and free from processed ingredients, is foundational to cellular health. Nutrients like vitamins, minerals, antioxidants, and amino acids are not just beneficial for the body in general—they are critical at the cellular level. For example, antioxidants neutralize free radicals, molecules that can damage cells and accelerate aging. Vitamins like B12 and magnesium are essential for mitochondrial function, while omega-3 fatty acids support cell membrane integrity and reduce inflammation.

Yet, nutrition alone cannot sustain cellular health if other areas—such as sleep, stress management, and exercise—are neglected. Chronic stress is one of the most significant contributors to cellular damage. Elevated levels of cortisol, the hormone associated with stress, can impair cellular repair mechanisms, increase inflammation, and lead to mitochondrial dysfunction. Sleep, meanwhile, is vital for cellular regeneration. Studies show that most tissue repair and detoxification processes occur during deep sleep, allowing cells to repair damage and regenerate.

Physical activity also plays a fundamental role in cellular health by stimulating mitochondrial biogenesis, the process through which cells produce more mitochondria. Exercise not only improves circulation, delivering oxygen and nutrients to cells, but also helps remove waste products from the body. Both high-intensity and low-intensity exercise contribute to cellular resilience, supporting cardiovascular health, reducing inflammation, and enhancing cognitive function.

Leveraging Ancient Wisdom and Modern Science

This book provides a comprehensive guide to natural methods for enhancing cellular function and restoring balance, blending ancient wisdom with modern science. Practices like meditation, grounding, and mindfulness are powerful tools for reducing stress and enhancing the body's natural healing abilities. Grounding, or direct physical contact with the earth, has been shown to reduce inflammation and improve sleep. Hydration, a simple but often overlooked component of health, supports cellular function, aids in detoxification, and helps maintain energy levels.

Emerging therapies like red light therapy, ozone therapy, and targeted nutritional supplements offer additional, science-backed ways to optimize cellular health. Red light therapy, for example, can penetrate deep into tissues, supporting mitochondrial function, reducing inflammation, and promoting tissue repair. Ozone therapy works by increasing oxygen levels and stimulating the immune system, making it especially useful for individuals with chronic conditions. Nutritional supplements like CoQ10, taurine, and glutathione provide essential support for mitochondrial health, cellular detoxification, and tissue repair.

Taking Responsibility for Our Health

The most empowering aspect of cellular health is realizing that we hold the keys to influencing it. While genetic factors are a part of our health story, the choices we make each day play a significant role in determining our health outcomes. The journey toward cellular wellness requires commitment and a willingness to take responsibility for our well-being. It isn't a quick fix, nor is it a "magic pill." Instead, it's a gradual, consistent process—a marathon, not a sprint—that requires us to make small, meaningful choices every day.

In the chapters that follow, we'll explore various aspects of cellular health, from the vital role of cellular energy and mitochondrial function to practical tools for reducing inflammation, enhancing detoxification, and supporting cellular repair. Chapter One will begin with the basics, exploring how our cells generate energy and how our daily choices—from what we eat to how we manage stress—impact this process. Each chapter builds upon the last, offering a layered approach that allows you to progressively incorporate these practices into your life.

A Call to Action

As we embark on this journey together, remember that every small step you take toward better health matters. Healing and optimizing cellular health isn't about drastic, overnight changes. It's about making one intentional choice at a time and building a foundation of resilience and vitality. The body's capacity to heal is extraordinary, and when we support our cells, we unlock that potential.

This book is your roadmap to harnessing the remarkable self-healing abilities within you. Embrace the process with patience, consistency, and a willingness to learn. Your journey to cellular wellness begins here. Remember, you don't have to take this journey alone, and every choice you make today is an investment in a healthier tomorrow. Let's begin with the foundational concept of cellular energy. By understanding how our cells produce and manage energy, we can set the stage for vibrant, lasting health—starting at the cellular level.

CHAPTER ONE

Understanding Cellular Energy

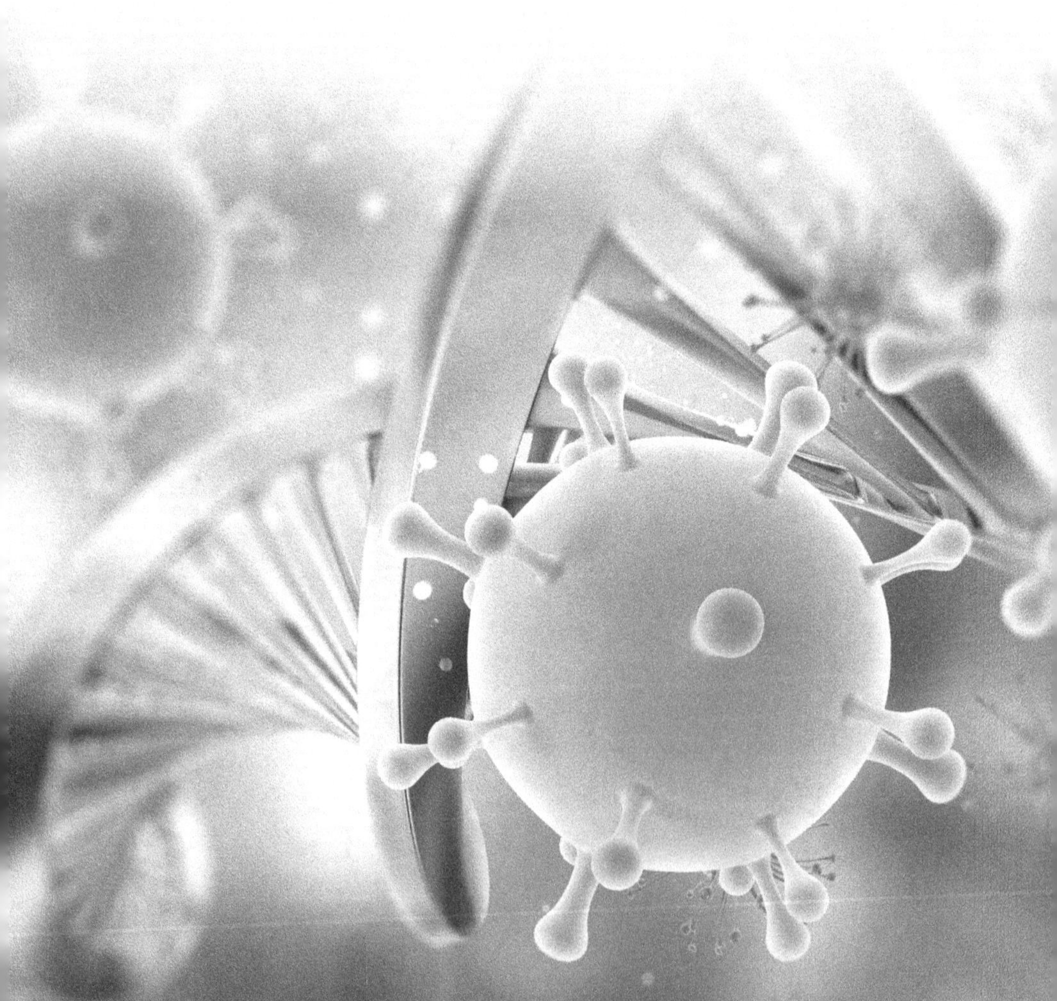

Albert Szent-Györgyi, a pioneer in cellular energy research, captured the essence of life with his statement, "Energy is the currency of life." This phrase perfectly expresses the crucial role energy plays in every biological function. Cellular energy is at the core of our ability to move, think, heal, and live. Without energy, the human body would cease to function, as every system relies on a continuous, efficient supply of energy to carry out essential tasks. Understanding how energy is produced, maintained, and distributed within our cells is fundamental to achieving optimal health, longevity, and vitality.

Cellular Energy (ATP) as the Foundation of Life

The molecule that provides cellular energy is adenosine triphosphate (ATP), often referred to as the "energy currency" of the cell. ATP consists of three phosphate groups, and the high-energy bonds between these phosphates store potential energy that is released to fuel the body's countless functions—from muscle contraction to nerve signaling to cellular repair. Every action in the body—whether conscious or unconscious—requires ATP. The production, storage, and use of ATP are central to cellular health and, by extension, our well-being. A single cell may contain millions of ATP molecules, and the human body regenerates its entire weight in ATP every day to keep up with demand.

ATP is primarily produced in the mitochondria, the powerhouse of the cell, through a process known as oxidative phosphorylation. To put this in perspective, imagine ATP as fuel in a car, with mitochondria functioning like the engine that transforms fuel into motion. Just as a car needs to refuel constantly to keep running, our cells need to continually regenerate ATP to sustain life. Mitochondria, therefore, play a vital role in converting the energy stored in food into a usable form that powers cellular functions.

The Mitochondria: Powerhouse of Cellular Energy

Mitochondria are often called the "powerhouses" of the cell, but their role extends beyond simply producing energy. Each cell in the human body contains hundreds, sometimes thousands, of mitochondria, depending on the energy needs of that cell. Cells in high-energy-demand organs, such as the heart, brain, and muscles, have especially high concentrations of mitochondria. Mitochondria convert nutrients from food—carbohydrates, fats, and proteins—into ATP through a complex series of biochemical reactions known as the electron transport chain (ETC), located in the inner mitochondrial membrane.

The process of cellular respiration begins with the breakdown of glucose (a sugar), fats, and proteins into smaller molecules like pyruvate and acetyl-CoA. Pyruvate, derived from carbohydrates, undergoes glycolysis in the cell's cytoplasm, where it is converted into acetyl-CoA, which then enters the mitochondria. Inside the mitochondria, these molecules enter the Krebs cycle (or citric acid cycle), generating high-energy molecules that feed into the electron transport chain. As electrons move along this chain, they release energy used to pump hydrogen ions across the mitochondrial membrane, creating a concentration gradient. This gradient powers ATP synthase, an enzyme that synthesizes ATP.

While this process may sound complex, it can be visualized like a hydro-electric dam, where the flow of water (electrons) generates energy by driving turbines (ATP synthase) to produce electricity (ATP). In mitochondria, the electron flow through the ETC powers the production of ATP, making this cycle the main energy source for nearly every function in the body. Any disruption in this energy flow can impair ATP production and affect every cell that depends on this energy.

Mitochondria and Cellular Metabolism: A Balancing Act

Beyond ATP production, mitochondria regulate cellular metabolism—the collection of chemical reactions that allow cells to grow, reproduce, and respond to environmental changes. In addition to energy production, mitochondria help manage reactive oxygen species (ROS), also known as free radicals, which are natural byproducts of cellular respiration. While ROS are essential for some cell signaling pathways, they can also damage cellular components, including DNA and proteins, when present in excess. Healthy mitochondria carefully balance ROS production and antioxidant defenses to prevent oxidative stress, which can damage cells.

When mitochondria function optimally, they efficiently produce ATP, minimize oxidative stress, and contribute to cellular health. However, when mitochondrial function is compromised—due to nutrient deficiencies, chronic stress, or toxin exposure—ATP production declines, leading to symptoms like fatigue, cognitive issues, and muscle weakness. Research in the Journal of Neuroscience has linked mitochondrial dysfunction to numerous age-related conditions, including Alzheimer's and cardiovascular disease. Supporting mitochondrial health is, therefore, essential for sustaining energy and long-term vitality.

How Chronic Inflammation and Insulin Resistance Disrupt Cellular Energy

Chronic inflammation is one of the major disruptors of cellular energy production. Inflammation is an ongoing immune response that damages mitochondria. According to research from The Lancet, inflammatory molecules called cytokines can interfere with the electron transport chain, reducing ATP output and increasing ROS production. This creates a vicious cycle: inflammation damages mitochondria, reducing ATP production, which in turn exacerbates inflammation and oxidative stress, further impairing cellular energy.

Insulin resistance—where cells become less responsive to the hormone insulin—also impairs ATP production. Insulin facilitates glucose entry into cells, providing the substrate for ATP production. When cells resist insulin, glucose cannot effectively enter, leading to reduced ATP production. Insulin resistance, as noted in the Journal of Endocrinology and Metabolism, not only decreases energy but also contributes to metabolic diseases like diabetes and obesity, placing further stress on mitochondria.

Think of mitochondria like high-performing athletes. Just as athletes need ideal conditions to perform—proper nutrition, hydration, and rest—mitochondria require a balanced environment to function optimally. Inflammation and insulin resistance are like persistent hurdles that interfere with mitochondria's "performance," leading to energy deficits that can contribute to chronic diseases and fatigue.

Natural Approaches to Optimizing Cellular Energy: Sunlight, Grounding, Exercise, and Breathing Techniques

While inflammation and insulin resistance disrupt mitochondrial function, nature offers powerful ways to restore balance and support cellular energy production. Sunlight, grounding, exercise, and breathing techniques are among these strategies, each not only enhancing ATP production but also contributing to overall health and resilience. We will explore each of these approaches in greater depth in later chapters, equipping you with a comprehensive understanding of how they can optimize cellular health.

Sunlight

Sunlight serves as a remarkable natural energizer. Exposure to ultraviolet (UV) light stimulates the production of vitamin D, which supports mitochondrial function by regulating calcium, an essential component for ATP synthesis. But beyond vitamin D, sunlight also delivers infrared light that penetrates cells and stimulates cytochrome c oxidase, a crucial enzyme in the electron transport chain, further boosting ATP production. Think of mitochondria as miniature solar panels, activated by sunlight to fuel energy production and enhance cellular health.

Grounding, or earthing, complements sunlight by offering antioxidant benefits. When we make direct contact with the Earth, we absorb free electrons that neutralize reactive oxygen species (ROS), reducing oxidative stress and protecting mitochondria from damage. This benefit, highlighted in the Journal of Environmental and Public Health, boosts ATP output. Imagine grounding as a way of "recharging" your body's natural battery, where electrons from the Earth help restore mitochondrial health and stabilize ATP production.

Exercise

Exercise is one of the most effective methods for supporting mitochondrial health. Physical activity promotes mitochondrial biogenesis—the creation of new mitochondria—thereby increasing the cell's capacity for ATP production. High-intensity interval training (HIIT) and strength training are particularly effective at stimulating mitochondrial growth. More mitochondria mean higher ATP availability, which translates to greater energy and vitality. Regular exercise also improves insulin sensitivity, enabling cells to more efficiently absorb glucose and produce ATP. Think of exercise as a workout for your mitochondria, strengthening their ability to generate energy and bolstering cellular resilience.

Breathing Techniques

Breathing techniques further reinforce cellular energy production by optimizing oxygen supply. Deep diaphragmatic breathing or pranayama enhances oxygen delivery to cells, which is crucial for efficient energy production. Oxygen serves as the final electron acceptor in the electron transport chain, a critical step in ATP synthesis. Studies show that controlled breathing reduces oxidative stress and improves mitochondrial efficiency. Visualize oxygen as the final component in a carefully constructed circuit, completing the flow of energy in cells. Controlled breathing fills your "energy circuit," maximizing oxygen levels to optimize ATP production.

These natural strategies—sunlight, grounding, exercise, and breathing techniques—are highly effective at restoring and supporting cellular energy production. Each practice nurtures mitochondrial health, helping our cells sustain energy levels and build resilience. As we explore these topics further in later chapters, you'll gain a deeper understanding of how to implement these practices for lasting vitality and well-being.

The Path to Cellular Energy Optimization

Understanding ATP and mitochondrial function is key to maintaining energy and health. By addressing disruptions like chronic inflammation and insulin resistance, and by adopting energy-enhancing practices like sunlight exposure, grounding, exercise, and deep breathing, you empower your body's ability to produce energy and foster resilience. Cellular vitality is within reach, and focusing on mitochondrial health unlocks our potential for a vibrant, healthy life.

Our cells are inherently made of energy, each vibrating at a specific frequency—measured in hertz—that is essential for sustaining life. This cellular frequency, typically between 60 to 70 hertz in healthy cells, facilitates communication between cells, enabling them to perform their functions efficiently. This vibration is not an abstract concept; it represents the electrical energy produced by mitochondria as they create ATP, the molecule that powers nearly every action in the body. When cellular energy depletes, cells cannot sustain their workload. The complex processes of repair, detoxification, and regeneration slow down, and systems within the body begin to weaken.

Imagine a battery slowly draining. At first, performance decreases, and you may experience vague symptoms like fatigue, brain fog, or mild discomfort. But if the energy depletion continues, it can lead to chronic conditions. As the energy deficit deepens, cells may enter a state of cellular senescence, where they no longer divide or contribute to tissue health. Eventually, without enough energy, cells may suffer irreversible damage and die, leading to tissue and organ dysfunction, and ultimately, disease.

To put it simply, think of cellular energy like the battery in a smartphone. When fully charged, your phone operates at peak performance, allowing you to access all its functions—calls, messages, apps, etc. But as the battery depletes, it slows down, and certain apps may not load properly—just like your cells struggle to perform essential functions when ATP levels drop. If the battery becomes critically low, the phone may shut down entirely, much like how cells can reach a point of no return if their energy needs aren't met. And just as regularly recharging your phone keeps it functioning, consistently supporting your cellular health with proper diet, exercise, sunlight, and sleep helps your cells maintain their energy balance and functionality.

This analogy underscores why optimizing cellular energy is so vital. By addressing factors that contribute to energy depletion—like inflammation and insulin resistance—and incorporating practices that recharge and protect cellular energy, we can sustain our health, prevent disease, and even slow down aging at the cellular level. As we explore these strategies in later chapters, you will see how they're not only essential for immediate well-being but also for ensuring long-term resilience and vitality.

CHAPTER TWO

Cellular Membrane Health

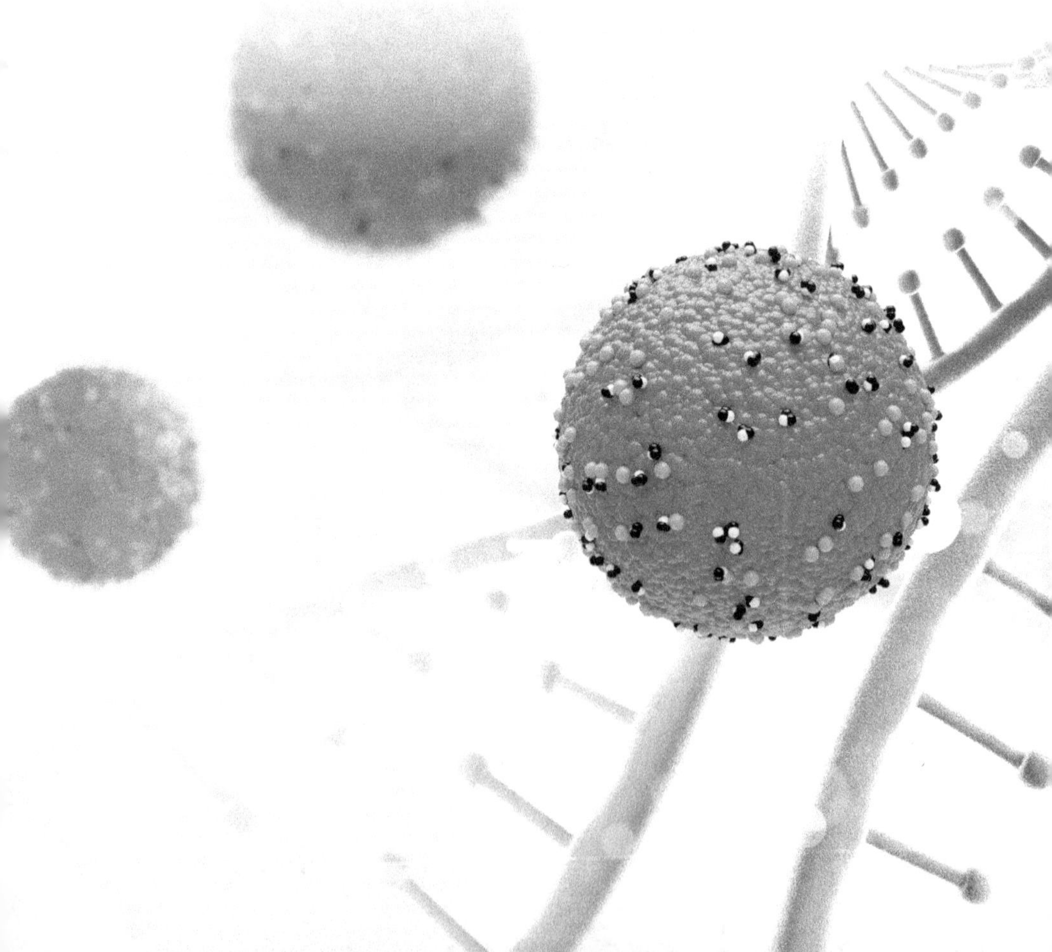

"A healthy outside starts from the inside." —Robert Urich

Robert Urich's quote, "A healthy outside starts from the inside," serves as a poignant reminder that our external health reflects what happens at the cellular level. The cell membrane, which protects and regulates each cell, plays a critical role in maintaining the health of our entire body. Its integrity is vital for cellular communication, nutrient absorption, and defense against external threats. Cell membranes are essential for cell health, acting as dynamic protective barriers that regulate the internal environment. They not only safeguard the cell's contents but also facilitate the selective transport of vital substances into and out of the cell. A chronically inflamed cell membrane may fail to let the good in or allow the bad out. Understanding the structure and function of cell membranes is crucial for supporting their health—and, by extension, our overall well-being and cellular vitality.

Structure of Cell Membranes

At the core of every cell membrane lies a phospholipid bilayer, a structural feature fundamental to its function. Each phospholipid molecule consists of a hydrophilic (water-attracting) head and two hydrophobic (water-repelling) tails. This amphipathic nature allows phospholipids to arrange themselves into two layers, with the heads facing outward toward the aqueous environment and the tails tucked away from it. This arrangement forms a semi-permeable membrane that allows for fluidity and flexibility, much like a well-designed fence that keeps out intruders while still letting the breeze flow through.

Embedded within this bilayer are various proteins, cholesterol, and carbohydrates, each contributing to the membrane's functionality. Integral proteins span the entire membrane and serve crucial roles in transport and communication, acting as channels or carriers for specific molecules. Think of these proteins as turnstiles at a concert; they ensure that only authorized guests can enter, which is essential for maintaining the integrity of the event (or, in this case, the cell). These proteins expedite the passage of ions and polar molecules, which cannot diffuse freely through the lipid bilayer due to their charge or size.

Peripheral proteins, located on the membrane's surface, provide structural support and participate in signaling pathways. They can interact with integral proteins and lipids, forming complexes essential for various cellular functions. Imagine these peripheral proteins as the security team surrounding the venue, ensuring everything runs smoothly and responding quickly if something unusual occurs.

Cholesterol is another vital component of cell membranes, strategically interspersed within the phospholipid bilayer. Cholesterol molecules help maintain membrane fluidity and stability, ensuring the membrane remains flexible yet robust enough to withstand changes in the external environment. This fluidity is essential for the effective functioning of membrane proteins and is crucial for cellular processes like endocytosis (the process of absorbing substances into the cell) and exocytosis (the process of releasing substances from the cell). Picture cholesterol as the lubricant in a well-oiled machine, allowing its parts to move smoothly and efficiently.

Carbohydrates are also present on the extracellular surface of the membrane, often attached to proteins (glycoproteins) or lipids (glycolipids). These carbohydrate chains form a protective layer known as the glycocalyx, which plays a pivotal role in cell recognition and communication. You can think of the glycocalyx as the signage and lighting outside a business, helping visitors identify the place and signaling that it's open for business. It is essential for immune responses, as it helps the immune system distinguish between the body's own cells (self) and foreign invaders (non-self), such as pathogens. The glycocalyx acts as a physical barrier, trapping pathogens and preventing them from reaching the cell membrane. Alterations in this protective layer can lead to autoimmune diseases, so optimizing it is vital for immune recognition, response, and overall cellular health.

The Function of Cell Membranes

Healthy cell membranes are crucial for numerous physiological processes. Their selective permeability allows certain substances to pass while blocking others, helping maintain homeostasis within the cell. For instance, small nonpolar molecules, such as oxygen and carbon dioxide, can easily diffuse across the membrane, much like a light breeze passing through a mesh screen. In contrast, larger or polar molecules, like glucose, require specific transport proteins to facilitate their entry—much like a key unlocking a door.

The membrane's ability to regulate the internal balance of ions and molecules is vital for processes such as cellular respiration, energy production, and metabolic functions. For example, the sodium-potassium pump actively transports sodium ions out of the cell while bringing potassium ions in, creating an electrochemical gradient essential for nerve impulse transmission and muscle contractions. Imagine this pump as a battery charger, ensuring the cell has the right amount of energy and resources to function effectively.

Moreover, cell membranes are involved in signal transduction, a process in which extracellular signals, such as hormones or growth factors, bind to receptors on the membrane surface. This binding induces conformational changes in the receptor, triggering a cascade of intracellular events that result in specific cellular responses. Disruption of this signaling pathway due to compromised membrane integrity can lead to various health issues, including hormonal imbalances and impaired immune responses. Think of this process as a telephone call: the receptor receives a message and transmits it to the rest of the cell, prompting it to take action.

Consequences of Impaired Membrane Health

When cell membranes suffer from chronic inflammation, their function can be significantly impaired. Inflammation alters membrane fluidity, leading to structural changes that weaken its barrier function. A compromised membrane may allow toxins and waste products to accumulate inside the cell, while also hindering the uptake of beneficial nutrients and hormones. It's like a blocked drain, where nutrients (water) cannot flow freely, leading to stagnation and subsequent problems.

Chronic inflammation creates a hostile cellular environment, often marked by increased oxidative stress. This stress can produce reactive oxygen species (ROS), which damage lipid components of the membrane through lipid peroxidation. Imagine ROS as rust forming on a metal surface; over time, this damage can lead to structural failure. As lipid peroxidation progresses, membranes can become "leaky," disrupting cellular homeostasis and signaling pathways.

Cells have a protective mechanism called the danger response, which activates when they detect threats like pathogens or stress. This response triggers protective pathways, including activating antioxidant systems and recruiting immune cells. However, persistent inflammation can dysregulate this response, leading to further dysfunction and making it harder for the cell to react properly to actual threats. It's like a smoke alarm that goes off too often—when there's a real fire, people might ignore it.

Impaired cell membranes can also affect immune function. Healthy membranes are crucial for detecting pathogens and initiating immune responses. Central to this process are proteins called major histocompatibility complex (MHC) molecules, which are found on the surface of our cells. MHC molecules act as "ID badges," helping the immune system distinguish between the body's own cells and foreign invaders like bacteria and viruses.

When a cell is infected or contains abnormal substances, MHC molecules display fragments of these intruders on the cell's surface. This alerts immune cells to the threat, enabling them to respond and combat the infection. MHC molecules play a key role in the immune system's ability to differentiate between "self" and "non-self," a distinction vital for maintaining health. If the cell membrane's integrity is compromised, the immune system may struggle to function properly, increasing susceptibility to infections.

Age-Related Changes in Membrane Health

As we age, cell membranes can become less fluid and more rigid due to factors like oxidative stress, inflammation, and dietary changes. This loss of membrane fluidity negatively affects nutrient transport, signaling, and overall cellular responsiveness, contributing to age-related health issues. Aging cell membranes are similar to old rubber bands—they lose their elasticity and can't stretch or bounce back as effectively.

Research has shown that lipid composition also changes with age, leading to an imbalance of fatty acids in the membrane. For example, the ratio of omega-3 to omega-6 fatty acids may shift unfavorably, promoting inflammation. This imbalance impairs the membrane's ability to adapt to environmental changes and reduces its effectiveness in nutrient uptake and waste removal.

The decline in membrane health is linked to chronic conditions such as cardiovascular disease and diabetes. For instance, atherosclerosis, which involves plaque buildup in the arteries, is associated with inflammation and oxidative damage to the endothelial cell membranes. This damage compromises the barrier function of blood vessels, leading to further cardiovascular complications.

Factors Affecting Membrane Health

Various lifestyle and environmental factors can negatively impact cell membrane health. Diet plays a significant role; consuming processed foods, unhealthy fats, and sugars can promote inflammation and oxidative stress. For example, trans fats and excessive omega-6 fatty acids can stiffen membranes, while a lack of omega-3 fatty acids reduces membrane fluidity. Think of your diet as the fuel for a vehicle—poor-quality fuel can lead to engine trouble.

Environmental toxins, such as heavy metals and pollutants, also disrupt membrane integrity. These toxins alter the membrane's structure and function, contributing to increased inflammation and cellular dysfunction. Chronic stress, combined with age-related changes, can exacerbate these issues, creating a cycle that further impairs cellular health.

Strategies to Support Cell Membrane Health

Several natural strategies can help support cell membrane health. Dietary choices play a crucial role in maintaining optimal membrane integrity. A balanced diet rich in whole foods, healthy fats, and antioxidants is essential. Key nutrients that contribute to healthy cell membranes include:

- **Omega-3 Fatty Acids:** Found in fatty fish (like salmon, mackerel, and sardines), flaxseeds, walnuts, and chia seeds, omega-3 fatty acids help maintain membrane fluidity and integrity. These healthy fats can reduce inflammation and oxidative stress, crucial for overall cellular health.

- **Phosphatidylcholine:** A vital component of cell membranes, found in eggs, soybeans, and sunflower seeds, phosphatidylcholine supports membrane integrity and cellular function.

- **Vitamin C:** An important antioxidant that protects cell membranes from oxidative damage, vitamin C is found in citrus fruits (like oranges and grapefruits), strawberries, kiwi, bell peppers, and broccoli.

- **Vitamin E**: Another key antioxidant, vitamin E helps prevent oxidative damage to membranes. Good sources include nuts (especially almonds and hazelnuts), seeds (like sunflower seeds), and healthy oils (such as olive oil and avocado oil).

- **Taurine**: Often called a "master osmolyte," taurine supports cellular health by stabilizing membranes and protecting cells from stress. It's found in meat, fish, and dairy products.

Importance of Hydration and Exercise

Hydration is essential for maintaining the health and functionality of cell membranes. Water is the primary component of bodily fluids and supports numerous physiological processes, including nutrient transport and waste removal. Adequate hydration ensures that nutrients can move into cells while helping to flush out metabolic waste products, maintaining a balanced internal environment crucial for cellular vitality. When hydration levels are optimal, cell membranes retain their fluidity and flexibility, enabling them to function effectively. Dehydration, however, increases the viscosity of cellular fluids, making it harder for substances to move across membranes. This thickening is similar to motor oil becoming too thick, which hinders engine performance. Without sufficient hydration, cells struggle to function properly, impacting overall health.

It's important to recognize that not all fluids hydrate equally. While water is the most effective hydrator, other beverages and foods can also contribute. For example, fruits and vegetables like cucumbers, watermelon, and oranges have high water content and provide vitamins and minerals that support cellular function. In contrast, excessive consumption of caffeinated or sugary beverages can lead to dehydration, as these drinks may act as diuretics or contribute to a calorie surplus without offering adequate hydration. Prioritizing water intake and hydrating foods is essential for maintaining cellular health.

Regular Exercise and Cell Membrane Health

Regular exercise is equally crucial for supporting cell membrane health. Physical activity improves blood circulation, which is vital for delivering nutrients and oxygen to cells while promoting the removal of metabolic waste products. Enhanced circulation ensures that cells receive the necessary resources to function optimally and regenerate effectively. Moreover, engaging in aerobic exercise, such as walking, running, or cycling, has anti-inflammatory effects that benefit cell membrane integrity. Research shows that exercise stimulates the production of anti-inflammatory cytokines and reduces pro-inflammatory markers, leading to a decrease in systemic inflammation.

Exercise also promotes the production of heat shock proteins (HSPs), which protect cells from stressors, including oxidative stress. These proteins stabilize cellular structures, including membranes, and improve cellular resilience. In this way, regular physical activity acts as a natural defense against the damaging effects of inflammation and oxidative stress, which can impair cell membrane function.

In addition to its direct effects on circulation and inflammation, exercise supports cardiovascular health. A well-functioning cardiovascular system is crucial for maintaining the flow of blood, nutrients, and oxygen throughout the body. This circulation is essential for all cellular activities, including those within cell membranes. For instance, aerobic exercise increases heart rate and promotes vascular health, ensuring that blood vessels remain flexible and responsive to the body's needs. Improved cardiovascular health enhances tissue oxygenation and the removal of carbon dioxide and waste products, supporting cellular homeostasis.

Incorporating regular physical activity into daily routines is simple and enjoyable. Brisk walks, cycling, or participating in sports or fitness classes can all be effective. The key is to find activities that encourage consistency. The Centers for Disease Control and Prevention (CDC) recommends at least 150 minutes of moderate-intensity aerobic activity each week, along with muscle-strengthening exercises on two or more days per week. Following these guidelines can significantly improve hydration, circulation, and overall cell membrane health.

Stress Management and Sleep Quality

Effective stress management is critical for maintaining optimal cellular function and overall health. Chronic stress can profoundly affect the body, particularly hormone levels, increasing inflammation and compromising the integrity of cell membranes. When we experience stress, the body activates the hypothalamic-pituitary-adrenal (HPA) axis, releasing stress hormones like cortisol. While cortisol is beneficial in short bursts, prolonged elevation due to chronic stress can lead to dysregulated immune responses and heightened inflammation.

High inflammation levels can disrupt cellular communication and impair cell membrane function. For example, chronic inflammation can decrease membrane fluidity, causing stiffness and impairing functionality. This dysfunction hinders the cell's ability to transport nutrients, eliminate waste, and respond to signaling molecules. Stress management techniques such as meditation and yoga can help reduce these effects by promoting relaxation and decreasing the body's overall stress load.

Mindfulness practices, including meditation and deep-breathing exercises, activate the body's relaxation response. Research in Health Psychology shows that regular mindfulness practice can significantly lower cortisol levels, fostering a balanced hormonal environment essential for membrane health. Yoga, in particular, enhances autonomic nervous system regulation, improving emotional resilience and reducing stress. The combination of physical movement, breath control, and meditation in yoga helps cultivate a sense of calm, supporting cellular health.

In addition to managing stress, quality sleep is paramount for cellular repair and regeneration. Sleep is a restorative process during which the body conducts vital maintenance, including repairing cellular membranes and clearing metabolic waste. Research shows that during sleep, the brain's glymphatic system activates, removing toxins that accumulate throughout the day. This detoxification is crucial for maintaining cellular homeostasis and preventing the buildup of harmful substances that can lead to inflammation and dysfunction.

Poor sleep quality disrupts these restorative processes, leading to negative effects on cellular health. Studies published in Sleep show that inadequate sleep increases inflammatory markers, compromising cell membrane integrity. Sleep deprivation has also been linked to weakened immune function and reduced stress resilience, creating a vicious cycle that perpetuates inflammation and undermines overall health.

To improve sleep quality, individuals should prioritize good sleep hygiene. Establishing a calming bedtime routine, reducing screen exposure before bed, and maintaining a consistent sleep schedule can significantly improve sleep. Additionally, creating a sleep-conducive environment—dark, cool, and quiet—can promote deeper, more restorative sleep.

The Role of Supplements in Supporting Membrane Health

In addition to dietary strategies, various supplements play a key role in supporting cell membrane health. These supplements can help enhance the integrity and function of cell membranes, which is crucial for overall cellular vitality and well-being.

Omega-3 Fatty Acids: Omega-3 fatty acids, commonly found in fish oil supplements, are essential fats that significantly improve membrane fluidity and reduce inflammation. The primary omega-3s—eicosapentaenoic acid (EPA) and docosahexaenoic acid (DHA)—integrate into cell membranes, helping maintain their flexibility and resilience. Research published in the *American Journal of Clinical Nutrition* indicates that higher omega-3 intake is linked to improved membrane fluidity, which enhances cellular communication and nutrient transport.

Omega-3 fatty acids also possess potent anti-inflammatory properties. Chronic inflammation can negatively affect cell membrane integrity, leading to various health issues. A systematic review in the *Journal of Lipid Research* found that omega-3 supplementation can lower inflammatory markers, making it particularly beneficial for individuals who don't consume enough omega-3-rich foods, such as fatty fish (salmon, mackerel), flaxseeds, and walnuts. For those with a diet low in omega-3s, supplementation can help reduce inflammation and support optimal cell membrane function, promoting overall health.

Phosphatidylcholine: Phosphatidylcholine, derived from lecithin, is another vital supplement for maintaining membrane integrity. It is a major component of cell membranes, playing a key role in maintaining their structure and fluidity. According to a study published in *Biochimica et Biophysica Acta*, phosphatidylcholine helps regulate the permeability of cell membranes, which is critical for cellular communication and transport.

Supplementing with phosphatidylcholine can support cellular function, especially for individuals with compromised membrane integrity due to dietary deficiencies or environmental stressors. *Research in the Journal of Nutrition* suggests that phosphatidylcholine supplementation can enhance liver function and support lipid metabolism, further emphasizing its importance for overall cellular health.

However, it is important to note that phosphatidylcholine (PTC) should be used for short-term supplementation, particularly until more is understood about its interaction with the gut microbiome. Gut bacteria metabolize phosphatidylcholine into trimethylamine (TMA), which can then be converted into trimethylamine N-oxide (TMAO). Elevated TMAO levels have been linked to an increased risk of heart disease. Therefore, monitoring gut health and microbiome composition is critical when considering long-term phosphatidylcholine supplementation, to minimize any potential risks while still supporting membrane integrity.

Taurine: Taurine, a sulfur-containing amino acid, is another important supplement for cellular health. It stabilizes cell membranes and helps maintain intracellular hydration, which is essential for optimal cell function. Taurine acts as an osmolyte, helping cells adapt to changes in their environment, such as variations in osmotic pressure. A study published in *Amino Acids* highlights taurine's role in protecting cells from oxidative stress and supporting cellular homeostasis.

Taurine supplementation can be especially beneficial for individuals exposed to chronic stressors, such as high-intensity exercise, illness, or environmental toxins. Research published in *Nutrients* suggests that taurine can enhance exercise performance and recovery by reducing muscle damage and inflammation. Given its protective effects on cell membranes, taurine is an essential supplement for individuals with increased cellular demands.

Antioxidants: Antioxidants, including vitamin C and vitamin E, play a crucial role in protecting cell membranes from oxidative damage. These nutrients work together to neutralize harmful free radicals, preserving membrane integrity and function.

Vitamin C is a water-soluble antioxidant that helps regenerate other antioxidants and protect against oxidative stress. According to a review in Free

Radical Biology and Medicine, vitamin C stabilizes cell membranes by reducing lipid peroxidation, a process that can cause cell damage.

Vitamin E, a fat-soluble antioxidant, is incorporated into the lipid bilayer of cell membranes, where it protects against oxidative damage by scavenging free radicals. Research in the *American Journal of Clinical Nutrition* demonstrates that adequate vitamin E levels are essential for maintaining cell membrane integrity and preventing lipid peroxidation, which can compromise cellular function.

Supplementing with these antioxidants is especially beneficial for individuals experiencing increased oxidative stress, due to factors like poor diet, environmental pollutants, or chronic illnesses. By supporting cellular health and membrane integrity, antioxidants help promote overall well-being and resilience against disease.

Supplements such as omega-3 fatty acids, phosphatidylcholine, taurine, and antioxidants are essential for maintaining healthy cell membranes. These nutrients not only enhance membrane fluidity and integrity but also offer protective effects against inflammation and oxidative damage. By incorporating these supplements into a balanced dietary approach, individuals can support optimal cellular function, promote resilience against disease, and enhance overall health.

Reducing Exposure to Environmental Toxins

Minimizing exposure to environmental toxins is essential for maintaining cell membrane health. Substances like heavy metals, pollutants, and certain chemicals can significantly disrupt the structure and function of cell membranes. Research shows that exposure to these toxins can lead to increased inflammation, oxidative stress, and cellular dysfunction, ultimately compromising overall health and increasing the risk of chronic diseases.

Understanding Environmental Toxins

Environmental toxins include a wide range of harmful substances, such as heavy metals (lead, mercury, and cadmium), persistent organic pollutants (POPs) like polychlorinated biphenyls (PCBs) and dioxins, and various industrial chemicals found in everyday products. These toxins can enter the body through ingestion, inhalation, and skin contact, accumulating over time and potentially causing harmful health effects.

For example, studies have shown that heavy metals can integrate into cellular membranes, interfering with their normal function. According to a review in Environmental Health Perspectives, heavy metals cause oxidative damage to lipids, proteins, and DNA, leading to cell death and impaired function. The accumulation of these toxins can reduce membrane fluidity, making cells more rigid and less responsive to physiological signals.

Choosing Organic Foods

One effective strategy to reduce exposure to harmful chemicals is choosing organic foods whenever possible. Organic farming practices limit the use of synthetic pesticides and fertilizers, which can leave harmful residues on conventionally grown produce. Research published in the *British Journal of*

Nutrition suggests that consuming organic produce is associated with lower levels of pesticide exposure, reducing the risk of health issues like neurodevelopmental disorders and certain cancers.

Organic foods often contain higher levels of antioxidants and nutrients, which help combat oxidative stress and inflammation caused by environmental toxins. According to the American Journal of Clinical Nutrition, a diet rich in fruits and vegetables, especially organic ones, can support the body's natural detoxification pathways and improve overall cellular health.

Opting for Safe Containers

In addition to dietary choices, the materials used to store food and beverages can also influence exposure to environmental toxins. Plastics, particularly those containing bisphenol A (BPA) and phthalates, are linked to endocrine disruption and other health concerns. These substances can leach into food and drinks, especially when exposed to heat or acidity.

Switching to glass or stainless-steel containers instead of plastic can help minimize this risk. Research in *Environmental Health Perspectives* shows that using BPA-free or non-plastic containers significantly reduces the levels of these harmful chemicals in the body. These materials are not only safer for food storage but also environmentally friendly, supporting sustainable practices.

Improving Indoor Air Quality

Indoor air quality plays a significant role in overall health, as many people spend a substantial amount of time indoors. Common indoor pollutants include volatile organic compounds (VOCs) from paints, cleaning products, and furniture, as well as mold, dust, and pet dander. Poor indoor air quality can exacerbate respiratory issues and contribute to systemic inflammation.

To improve indoor air quality, regular assessments and improvements are essential. Using air purifiers with HEPA filters can effectively reduce airborne particles, including allergens and toxins. Proper ventilation—such as opening windows or using exhaust fans—can help disperse harmful substances and bring in fresh air. A study in the *Journal of Environmental Health* found that improving ventilation significantly reduced indoor air pollutants and improved respiratory health.

Incorporating indoor plants can also enhance air quality. Certain plants, like spider plants and peace lilies, are known to absorb harmful chemicals and improve oxygen levels, fostering a healthier environment.

By actively reducing exposure to environmental toxins through mindful dietary choices, safe food storage practices, and improved indoor air quality, individuals can support their cell membrane health and overall cellular function. This proactive approach is vital not only for maintaining cellular integrity but also for boosting resilience against chronic diseases and promoting long-term well-being. As we create a healthier environment for our cells, we empower ourselves to thrive, fostering vitality that radiates from the cellular level to every aspect of our lives.

Conclusion

Cell membrane health is foundational to overall cellular vitality. By understanding the importance of membranes and implementing natural strategies to support their integrity, individuals can significantly enhance their health and well-being. A balanced diet, regular exercise, effective stress management, and quality sleep all contribute to maintaining healthy cell membranes, allowing cells to function optimally.

When cell membranes operate effectively, they can manage the intake of beneficial substances and efficiently eliminate toxins. Prioritizing cell membrane health today can lead to substantial benefits in the years to come, enabling individuals to lead vibrant, energetic lives. By investing in the health of our cell membranes, we promote resilience against disease and enhance our body's ability to thrive.

As we've explored the critical role of cell membrane health in maintaining cellular integrity and function, it becomes clear that the environment surrounding our cells—the "cellular terrain"—is equally important. Just as healthy cell membranes facilitate nutrient transport and waste elimination, a balanced cellular terrain supports optimal cellular function and resilience against disease.

In the next chapter, we'll dive deeper into the concept of cellular terrain health, examining how factors such as nutrition, hydration, and lifestyle impact the terrain—and, in turn, our overall health and vitality. Understanding how to optimize our cellular environment is key to empowering our cells to thrive and promoting long-lasting health.

CHAPTER THREE

The Importance of Cellular Terrain

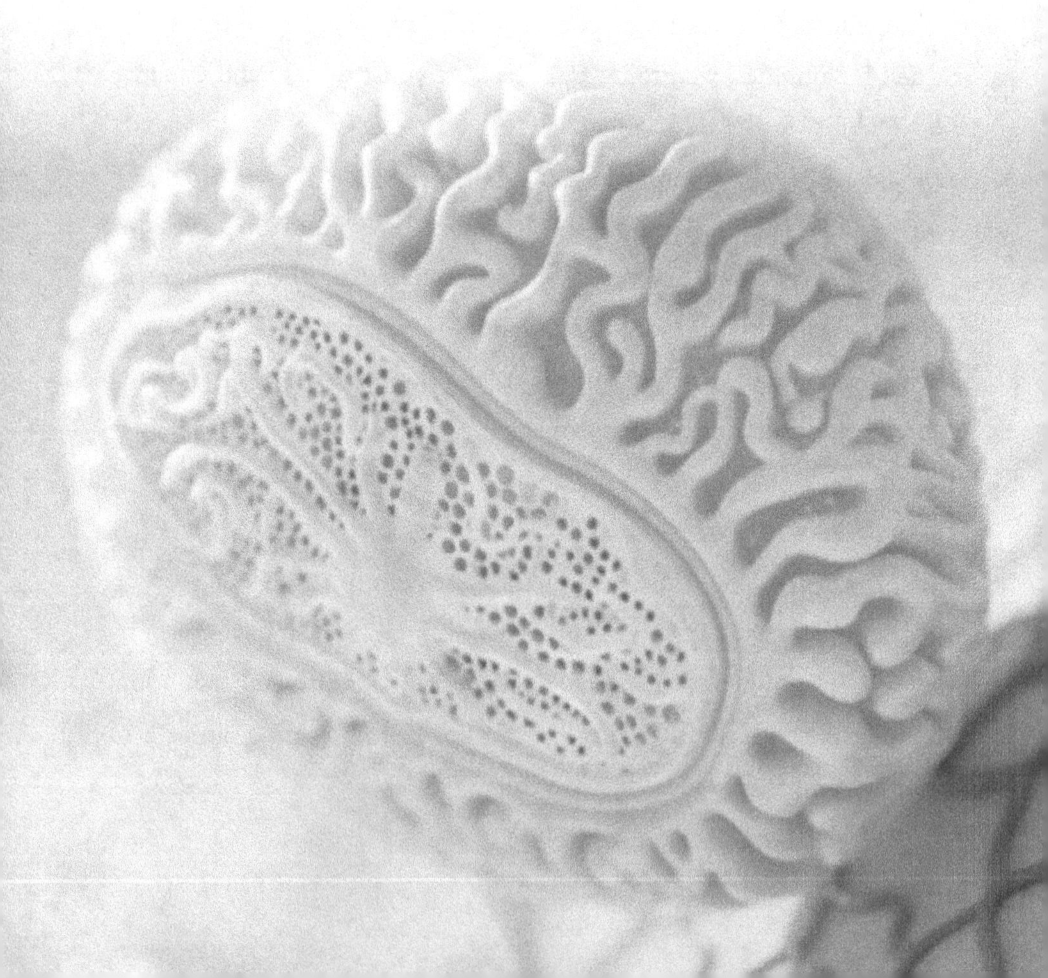

"Terrain matters more than the germ." —Antoine Béchamp

Antoine Béchamp's quote, "Terrain matters more than the germ," challenges the widely accepted belief that diseases are solely caused by pathogens like bacteria and viruses. Instead, Béchamp emphasized the significance of the body's internal environment—our "terrain"—in determining whether these germs can thrive and cause illness. The state of our cellular terrain—the environment surrounding our cells—is crucial for overall health and the body's ability to resist disease. In this chapter, we will explore the role of the extracellular matrix (ECM) in cellular health, detoxification strategies for maintaining a clean cellular environment, and the critical connection between gut health and the cellular terrain.

The Extracellular Matrix: A Foundation for Cellular Health

The cellular terrain is primarily defined by the extracellular matrix (ECM), a complex network that provides both structural and biochemical support to surrounding cells. Think of the ECM as the soil in a garden: just as healthy soil nourishes plants and enables them to grow, a healthy ECM provides the environment necessary for cells to function properly. The ECM is composed of various proteins, glycoproteins, and polysaccharides that form a scaffold for tissue architecture, facilitate intercellular communication, and support nutrient transport. The health of the ECM is crucial, as it directly influences how well cells can function, repair themselves, and respond to external signals.

Key Components of the Extracellular Matrix

The ECM consists of several essential elements that play a critical role in maintaining cellular function and overall tissue integrity:

- Collagen is the most abundant protein in the ECM, serving as a fibrous framework that provides strength and structure to various tissues, including skin, bones, and cartilage. You can think of collagen as the beams and supports in a building, which give the structure its shape and stability.

- Elastin is another key protein, enabling tissues to stretch and return to their original shape—similar to a rubber band. This elasticity is particularly important in organs that require flexibility, such as the lungs, which expand during breathing, and blood vessels, which need to adjust to changes in blood flow and pressure.

- Proteoglycans are molecules made up of a core protein with long chains of glycosaminoglycans (GAGs) attached. These structures are essential for retaining water and maintaining the hydration of the ECM, which is vital for cell signaling and nutrient transport. Think of proteoglycans as sponges within the ECM, soaking up water and helping to keep the environment around the cells moist and nutrient-rich.

- Glycoproteins are proteins with carbohydrate chains attached to them. These molecules play a significant role in cell adhesion, signaling, and regulating various cellular activities. You could think of glycoproteins as "sticky tape" that helps hold things together, anchoring cells in place and enabling communication between them—similar to how people use words to interact and convey messages.

The Role of the ECM in Cellular Function

The ECM acts not only as a physical scaffold but also as a reservoir for growth factors and cytokines, which are essential for cellular communication and immune responses. A healthy ECM enables cells to receive the signals necessary for repair, regeneration, and detoxification. In contrast, when the ECM is compromised due to toxins, inflammation, or oxidative stress, these processes are disrupted, leading to cellular dysfunction and disease.

For example, a buildup of toxins in the ECM can interfere with a cell's ability to detoxify itself. This accumulation creates a hostile environment, reducing the cell's energy production and its capacity for repair. It's like a factory that cannot operate efficiently because its machines are clogged with dust and debris; without proper cleaning and maintenance, productivity drops. Chronic inflammation—often driven by poor diet, stress, and environmental pollutants—only exacerbates the issue, leading to breakdowns in cellular communication and impaired immune responses.

Maintaining a healthy cellular terrain is about creating a clean, balanced environment where cells can thrive. When the terrain is compromised, it's much harder for cells to perform their essential functions, making them more susceptible to disease. By promoting a healthy ECM, we support optimal cellular function, detoxification, and repair, enhancing overall health and disease resistance.

Detoxification: Essential Strategies for a Healthy Cellular Environment

Detoxification is the body's innate process of eliminating toxins and waste products from cells and tissues, playing a vital role in overall health. In today's world, the cellular terrain can easily become overwhelmed by environmental pollutants, processed foods, and chronic stress, underscoring the need for effective natural detoxification strategies. These approaches are essential for maintaining a clean and healthy environment around our cells, ensuring they function optimally.

One of the most powerful methods for promoting detoxification and enhancing cellular health is intermittent fasting (IF). This practice has gained significant attention for its ability to trigger autophagy, a natural cellular process where damaged components, including toxins and dysfunctional organelles, are broken down and removed. Research published in *Cell Metabolism* confirms that this cleansing process significantly reduces oxidative stress, which can compromise the integrity of the extracellular matrix (ECM). During fasting periods, the body shifts from using glucose to burning fat for fuel, leading to the production of ketones. These ketones not only provide an alternative energy source but also act as protective agents, shielding cells from inflammation and oxidative damage. Think of intermittent fasting as scheduling a dedicated cleaning day for your body; it allows cells to focus on repair and rejuvenation, rather than digestion. Furthermore, intermittent fasting has been shown to improve insulin sensitivity and enhance mitochondrial function, further supporting a healthy cellular terrain.

Another effective detoxification strategy is grounding (or earthing), which involves direct contact with the Earth's surface—such as walking barefoot on grass or sand. This simple yet profound practice helps reduce inflammation and oxidative stress by neutralizing harmful free radicals. According to a study in the *Journal of Environmental and Public Health*, grounding facilitates the absorption of electrons from the Earth, which act as natural antioxidants, mitigating oxidative stress. Think of grounding as reconnecting your body to a natural power source; it replenishes your system and dissipates excess energy that can lead to inflammation. By lowering inflammation, grounding helps cleanse the ECM and promotes cellular repair. Additionally, it enhances circulation, further supporting the removal of toxins from the ECM, and has shown promise in reducing markers of inflammation and improving immune function.

Red light therapy, also known as photobiomodulation, is another innovative approach that supports detoxification and terrain health. This non-invasive treatment exposes the body to specific wavelengths of light, typically in the red and near-infrared spectrum. Research indicates that red light therapy enhances cellular energy production by stimulating the mitochondria, improving cellular metabolism and function. Additionally, red light therapy promotes detoxification by increasing lymphatic flow and circulation, helping to remove waste products and toxins from the body. The anti-inflammatory effects of red light therapy also support healing processes within the ECM, creating a more conducive environment for cellular repair and regeneration. Think of red light therapy as a revitalizing boost that encourages your cells to operate at peak efficiency while supporting the body's natural detoxification pathways.

Pulsed Electromagnetic Field (PEMF) therapy is another valuable tool for detoxification and cellular health. This therapy uses low-frequency electromagnetic fields to promote cellular function and enhance the body's natural detoxification processes. Research shows that PEMF therapy can improve circulation, reduce inflammation, and enhance lymphatic fluid flow, which are all crucial for toxin removal. By stimulating cellular metabolism and energy production, PEMF therapy supports the body's ability to detoxify more effectively. Imagine PEMF therapy as a gentle vibration that helps shake loose toxins and waste products, facilitating their removal while promoting overall cellular health.

Proper hydration is a cornerstone of effective detoxification. Water plays a critical role in flushing out toxins and metabolic waste products that accumulate in the extracellular matrix. Research in *The American Journal of Physiology* emphasizes that adequate hydration supports the kidneys and liver in their detoxification processes, ultimately reducing the burden on individual cells. Picture hydration as ensuring a continuous supply of clean water flowing into a reservoir; without it, toxins can accumulate, creating a stagnant and unhealthy environment. Additionally, water fasting—abstaining from food while consuming only water—can further enhance detoxification by allowing the body to prioritize cellular repair over digestion. This practice stimulates autophagy and promotes the elimination of toxins, leading to improved cellular function and heightened energy production.

Infrared saunas represent another effective approach to detoxification. By using infrared light to heat the body from the inside out, these saunas promote sweating, which assists in the elimination of toxins. Sweating is one of the body's primary mechanisms for detoxification, and infrared saunas are particularly effective at stimulating sweat production. A study in *The Journal of Environmental and Public Health* found that infrared saunas help remove heavy metals and other environmental toxins from the body, effectively cleansing the extracellular matrix and alleviating oxidative stress. Think of using an infrared sauna as offering your body a thorough detoxifying steam clean; it helps flush out impurities and rejuvenate internal systems. Regular sauna use has been associated with improved circulation, enhanced immune function, and strengthened natural detoxification pathways.

Incorporating a diet rich in detoxifying foods is equally essential for supporting the body's detoxification processes. Cruciferous vegetables, such as broccoli and kale, contain compounds like sulforaphane that bolster the body's ability to detoxify harmful substances. Research published in *The Journal of Nutrition* shows that sulforaphane activates detoxification enzymes in the liver, aiding in the purification of the cellular terrain. Other beneficial detoxifying foods include garlic, which provides sulfur compounds that support liver detoxification; beets, rich in betalains that reduce inflammation; and turmeric, known for its powerful anti-inflammatory and antioxidant properties. Including these foods in your diet is like providing high-quality fuel for a car; it helps the body operate efficiently while reducing the toxic load in the ECM and promoting cellular health.

The Connection Between Gut Health and Cellular Terrain

The health of the gut microbiome—the trillions of bacteria, viruses, and fungi residing in the digestive system—plays a critical role in maintaining the cellular terrain. The gut and extracellular matrix (ECM) are closely interconnected, as the gut microbiome influences inflammation, detoxification, and nutrient absorption, all of which affect the health of the ECM and overall cellular function.

Gut Barrier Integrity

The gut lining serves as a barrier, preventing harmful substances like toxins and pathogens from entering the bloodstream. When this barrier is compromised—a condition known as "leaky gut"—harmful substances can leak into the bloodstream, leading to systemic inflammation. Research published in *Gut Microbes* shows that leaky gut is associated with chronic inflammation, autoimmune diseases, and metabolic dysfunction, all of which negatively impact the cellular terrain. Imagine the gut lining as a fence around a garden: if the fence is broken, weeds and pests can invade, damaging the plants inside. A healthy gut barrier is essential for maintaining the integrity of the ECM, as it prevents the accumulation of toxins and inflammatory molecules that can damage cells.

Microbiome Diversity

A diverse gut microbiome is crucial for supporting immune function, reducing inflammation, and promoting detoxification. According to research in *Nature Reviews Immunology*, the gut microbiome plays a key role in regulating the immune system and controlling inflammation. A diverse microbiome produces short-chain fatty acids (SCFAs), such as butyrate, which have anti-inflammatory properties and help maintain the gut lining's integrity. Think of a diverse microbiome as a community of gardeners working together to keep the garden healthy—each contributing uniquely to prevent disease and promote growth. Supporting a healthy gut microbiome through a diet rich in prebiotics (fiber from fruits and vegetables) and fermented foods (like yogurt and sauerkraut) can enhance microbiome diversity and support gut health.

Gut-Brain Axis

The gut and brain are interconnected through the gut-brain axis, a communication network linking the central nervous system to the digestive system. The health of the gut microbiome can directly influence brain function, mood, and cognitive performance. Research in *Psychoneuroendocrinology* shows that a disrupted gut microbiome is associated with increased inflammation, which can impair brain function and contribute to neurodegenerative diseases. A healthy gut ensures proper communication between the brain and cells throughout the body, supporting optimal immune, nervous, and detoxification responses.

Nutrient Absorption

The gut is responsible for absorbing nutrients from food, which are then used to support cellular repair, energy production, and detoxification. Poor gut health can impair nutrient absorption, leading to deficiencies that negatively affect the cellular terrain. For instance, deficiencies in vitamins C and E, as well as glutathione, can compromise the body's ability to neutralize free radicals and protect the ECM from oxidative damage, as noted in The American Journal of Clinical Nutrition.

Probiotics are beneficial bacteria that support gut health by improving the balance of the microbiome, promoting digestion, and reducing inflammation. A study in Frontiers in *Microbiology* indicates that probiotics can help repair the gut barrier and enhance detoxification processes. By fostering a healthy gut, probiotics contribute to a supportive ECM and optimize cellular function.

Conclusion: Prioritizing Terrain Health for Optimal Cellular Function

The concept of terrain health is fundamental to understanding overall body health. A clean and balanced cellular environment not only influences detoxification and immune responses but also plays a crucial role in cellular communication and energy production. By maintaining a healthy extracellular matrix, supporting detoxification processes, and prioritizing gut health, we create an optimal terrain where cells can thrive.

As we explore these foundational concepts, it's essential to recognize how terrain health directly intersects with chronic inflammation and insulin resistance—two conditions that are increasingly prevalent in modern lifestyles and can profoundly affect cellular function and overall health. In the next chapter, we will examine the mechanisms behind chronic inflammation and insulin resistance, exploring how they develop, their impact on cellular terrain, and strategies to mitigate their effects for improved health and vitality.

CHAPTER FOUR

Chronic Inflammation and Insulin Resistance

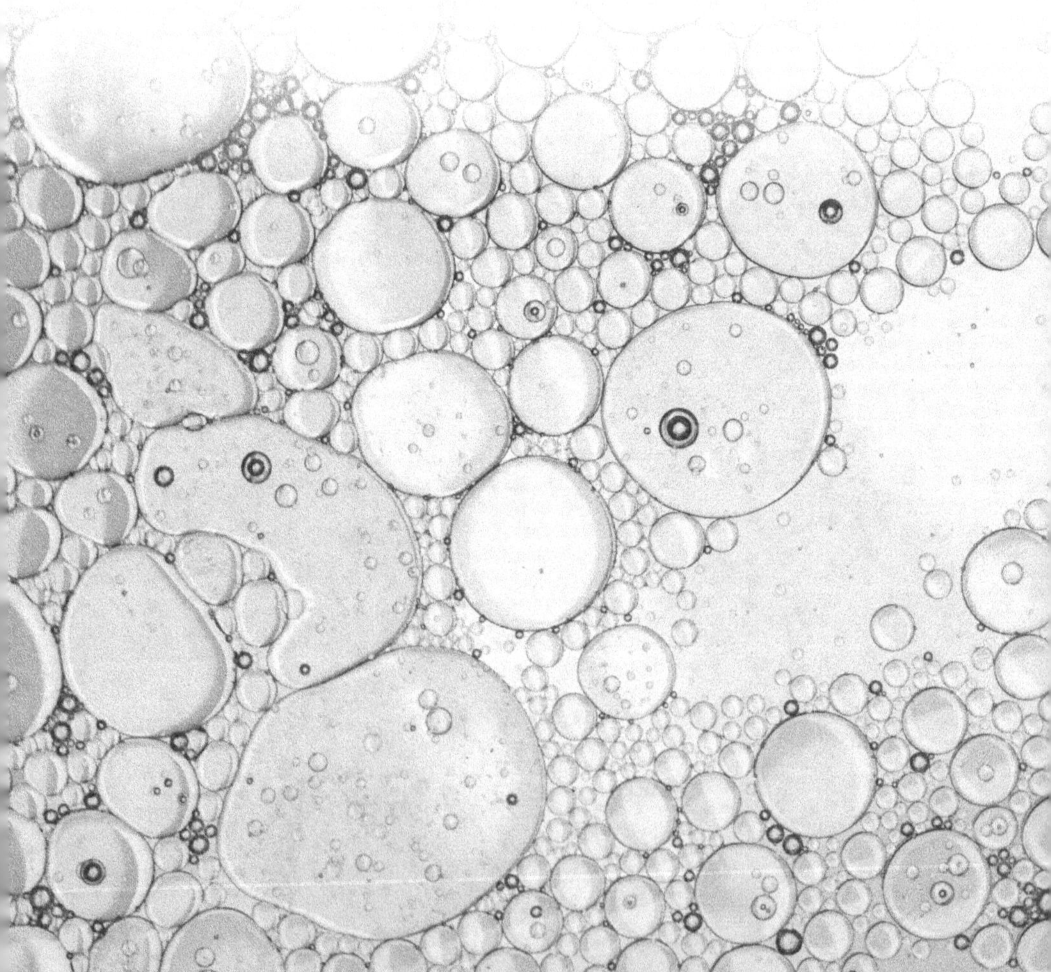

"Inflammation is the silent enemy." —Dr. Mark Hyman

Dr. Mark Hyman's powerful quote, "Inflammation is the silent enemy," underscores the often-hidden but profoundly destructive nature of chronic inflammation. It lurks beneath the surface, gradually eroding cellular function and contributing to a range of chronic diseases, from diabetes and heart disease to neurodegenerative conditions. When inflammation becomes chronic, it disrupts the body's natural balance, causing significant harm at the cellular level. This chapter explores the damaging effects of chronic inflammation on cellular health, the impact of insulin resistance on mitochondrial function, and the dietary and lifestyle strategies that can reduce inflammation and improve insulin sensitivity.

The Damaging Effects of Chronic Inflammation on Cellular Health

Inflammation is a natural immune response to injury or infection. In the short term, it helps the body heal by isolating the threat and initiating repair. However, when inflammation becomes chronic—often due to poor diet, stress, environmental toxins, and lack of physical activity—it becomes destructive. Chronic inflammation gradually damages tissues, disrupts cellular communication, and impairs the body's ability to heal itself. On a cellular level, chronic inflammation produces excessive free radicals, leading to oxidative stress that damages cell membranes, DNA, and mitochondria.

A study published in *The Journal of Clinical Investigation* shows that chronic inflammation increases the production of pro-inflammatory molecules like cytokines, which interfere with normal cellular function and promote the development of chronic diseases, including cardiovascular disease, diabetes, and cancer. The cells most affected are those with high metabolic activity, such as immune cells, muscle cells, and neurons. In these cells, inflammation impairs energy production, leading to cellular dysfunction, fatigue, and the accumulation of cellular waste. Over time, this can contribute to conditions like chronic fatigue syndrome, fibromyalgia, and neurodegenerative disorders such as Alzheimer's disease.

Furthermore, chronic inflammation disrupts the extracellular matrix (ECM), which is the cellular framework that supports and nourishes cells. When the ECM is damaged, it can no longer regulate nutrient flow, remove waste, or facilitate communication between cells. This impairs detoxification and cellular repair. The result is a vicious cycle where inflammation damages the ECM, and a compromised ECM further exacerbates inflammation. In short, chronic inflammation weakens cellular defenses, disrupts mitochondrial function, and impairs the body's ability to maintain homeostasis. Addressing chronic inflammation through diet, lifestyle, and specific anti-inflammatory practices is crucial for restoring cellular health and preventing long-term damage.

Understanding How Insulin Resistance Disrupts Cellular and Mitochondrial Function

Insulin is a hormone produced by the pancreas that helps cells absorb glucose from the bloodstream to produce energy. When cells become resistant to insulin, they can no longer effectively absorb glucose, leading to elevated blood sugar levels. Over time, insulin resistance impairs mitochondrial function, reduces energy production, and contributes to the development of chronic diseases like type 2 diabetes, obesity, and cardiovascular disease.

Insulin resistance primarily affects muscle, liver, and fat cells. Under normal conditions, insulin triggers the uptake of glucose, which is then used to produce ATP (adenosine triphosphate) in the mitochondria. However, in insulin-resistant cells, glucose uptake is impaired, resulting in lower ATP production and higher circulating blood glucose levels. A study published in *The Journal of Endocrinology* found that insulin resistance disrupts mitochondrial function by limiting the availability of glucose, the primary fuel source for energy production.

Mitochondria are the energy factories of the cell, and when deprived of glucose, their ability to produce ATP is compromised. This leads to cellular fatigue, impaired detoxification, and increased susceptibility to oxidative stress. Over time, oxidative stress damages mitochondrial DNA, further impairing energy production and accelerating cellular decline. Additionally, insulin resistance promotes chronic inflammation by triggering the release of pro-inflammatory cytokines from fat cells (adipocytes). These cytokines create a state of low-grade inflammation throughout the body, which further damages mitochondria and impairs cellular function. This creates a feedback loop in which insulin resistance and inflammation perpetuate each other, leading to a progressive decline in cellular health.

Research published in *Diabetes Care* suggests that reversing insulin resistance through diet and lifestyle interventions can restore mitochondrial function, reduce inflammation, and improve overall cellular health. By improving insulin sensitivity, cells can once again absorb glucose efficiently, produce adequate ATP, and detoxify harmful substances.

Symptoms of Chronic Inflammation and Insulin Resistance

Chronic inflammation and insulin resistance can manifest through a range of symptoms that significantly impact daily life. Recognizing these signs is crucial for early intervention and effective management.

Symptoms of Chronic Inflammation may include:

- Persistent fatigue and low energy levels
- Joint pain and stiffness, often worsening after periods of inactivity
- Frequent infections or illnesses due to a weakened immune response
- Skin issues, such as rashes, acne, or eczema
- Digestive problems, including bloating, gas, or irritable bowel syndrome (IBS)

Symptoms of Insulin Resistance can include:

- Increased hunger and cravings, particularly for sugary or carbohydrate-rich foods
- Weight gain, especially around the abdomen
- Difficulty losing weight despite diet and exercise efforts
- Fatigue, particularly after meals
- Dark patches of skin (acanthosis nigricans), often seen in body creases such as the neck and armpits

Understanding these symptoms can help readers identify potential health issues early, encouraging proactive steps to improve their health.

Dietary and Lifestyle Changes for Chronic Inflammation and Insulin Resistance

To combat chronic inflammation and insulin resistance, implementing specific dietary and lifestyle changes is essential.

Dietary Changes:

- **Adopt an Anti-Inflammatory Diet:** Focus on whole foods rich in antioxidants, healthy fats, and fiber to reduce inflammation and improve insulin sensitivity. Foods like fruits, vegetables, whole grains, and lean proteins should be staples in the diet.

- **Incorporate Omega-3 Fatty Acids:** Omega-3s, found in fatty fish (salmon, mackerel) and plant sources (flaxseeds, chia seeds), have powerful anti-inflammatory properties. They help reduce pro-inflammatory cytokines and support mitochondrial function.

- **Limit Processed Foods and Sugars:** Reducing intake of refined carbohydrates and sugars can decrease inflammation and improve insulin sensitivity. Highly processed foods contribute to insulin resistance and should be replaced with whole foods.

- **Choose Low Glycemic, High-Protein Foods:** Emphasizing foods that are low on the glycemic index helps maintain stable blood sugar levels. Lean proteins (chicken, turkey, legumes) should be included to enhance satiety and support muscle mass.

Engaging in regular physical activity is vital for reducing inflammation and improving insulin sensitivity. Exercise plays a multifaceted role in promoting overall health, especially concerning chronic inflammation and metabolic function. Aerobic activities such as walking, running, and cycling are particularly effective for enhancing cardiovascular health. These activities increase heart rate and blood circulation, improving oxygen delivery to tissues and helping eliminate metabolic waste products. Research consistently shows that aerobic exercise lowers pro-inflammatory cytokine levels, mitigating inflammation throughout the body.

Furthermore, aerobic exercise significantly improves insulin sensitivity by enhancing the body's ability to utilize glucose. Regular exercise makes muscle cells more responsive to insulin, improving glucose uptake from the bloodstream. This process is like priming a sponge to absorb water: the more you exercise, the more effectively your body handles blood sugar levels.

In addition to aerobic exercise, strength training is essential for building muscle mass and increasing glucose uptake. Resistance exercises such as weightlifting or bodyweight workouts stimulate muscle growth. Increased muscle mass is beneficial because muscle cells require more glucose for energy, which helps lower overall blood sugar levels. Strength training also promotes the release of growth factors that support muscle repair and regeneration, contributing to better metabolic health. It can also increase resting metabolic rate, allowing the body to burn more calories even at rest.

Regular exercise promotes the release of endorphins, the body's natural mood enhancers. These chemicals can elevate feelings of well-being and reduce pain perception. Exercise-induced endorphin release can lead to a more positive mindset, helping to counteract the mental fatigue often associated with chronic inflammation and stress.

Prioritize Sleep

Quality sleep is essential for regulating inflammation and maintaining insulin sensitivity. During sleep, the body undergoes critical restorative processes, including tissue repair and hormone regulation. Research shows that inadequate sleep raises levels of pro-inflammatory cytokines, worsening insulin resistance and contributing to metabolic dysfunction. Studies have found that individuals who consistently sleep less than seven hours per night exhibit increased markers of inflammation and impaired glucose tolerance.

To improve sleep quality, it's important to establish a consistent sleep routine. Going to bed and waking up at the same time each day helps regulate the body's internal clock and promotes better sleep patterns. Creating a restful sleep environment—characterized by a cool, dark, and quiet room—can also significantly enhance sleep quality. Limiting screen time before bed and avoiding stimulants like caffeine or nicotine in the evening are essential steps for ensuring restful sleep.

Practicing relaxation techniques before bedtime, such as reading or taking a warm bath, can further improve sleep quality. Quality sleep isn't just about duration; it's about the restorative processes that occur during deep sleep stages, which are vital for cellular repair and regeneration.

Managing stress is crucial, as chronic stress is a major contributor to both inflammation and insulin resistance. When the body is under stress, it produces cortisol, a hormone that, while helpful in short bursts, can have adverse effects when elevated over prolonged periods. Chronic high levels of cortisol promote the release of inflammatory markers and can exacerbate insulin resistance, creating a vicious cycle that further impairs metabolic health.

Implementing stress-reduction techniques is essential for counteracting the negative effects of stress on cellular health. Mindfulness meditation has been shown to lower cortisol levels and promote a sense of calm and clarity. This practice encourages individuals to focus on the present moment, reducing anxiety and stress while fostering a relaxed state of mind. Even a few minutes of mindfulness each day can have a profound impact on overall well-being.

Yoga is another effective stress-management technique that combines physical movement, breath control, and meditation. Research indicates that yoga can reduce inflammation and improve insulin sensitivity, making it a valuable addition to any health regimen. The gentle stretching and strengthening of muscles during yoga not only enhance physical well-being but also promote mental relaxation and emotional stability.

Deep-breathing exercises are a simple yet effective way to manage stress and lower cortisol levels. By focusing on slow, controlled breathing, individuals can activate the parasympathetic nervous system, which helps counteract the body's stress response. This practice promotes relaxation, reduces anxiety, and supports a balanced immune response.

Incorporating regular physical activity, prioritizing quality sleep, and managing stress through various techniques are all essential lifestyle changes that can combat chronic inflammation and insulin resistance. By taking a proactive approach to these areas, individuals can significantly enhance their overall health, improve cellular function, and promote long-term vitality.

Supplements for Chronic Inflammation and Insulin Sensitivity

In addition to dietary and lifestyle changes, certain supplements can play a crucial role in combating chronic inflammation and improving insulin sensitivity, ultimately benefiting cellular health. These supplements target the underlying causes of inflammation and insulin resistance, promoting a more balanced physiological state.

Chromium

Chromium is an essential trace mineral that enhances insulin sensitivity and improves glucose metabolism. It plays a critical role in the metabolism of carbohydrates, fats, and proteins by amplifying the effects of insulin. Research published in *Nutrition Research* suggests that chromium supplementation can help improve blood sugar control in individuals with insulin resistance by enhancing insulin receptor function, making cells more responsive to insulin. Think of chromium as a key that unlocks the door to cells, allowing glucose to enter more easily and fuel cellular functions. A deficiency in chromium may impair insulin signaling, exacerbating issues related to chronic inflammation and insulin resistance.

Carnitine is an amino acid derivative essential for fatty acid metabolism and mitochondrial function. It transports long-chain fatty acids into the mitochondria, where they are oxidized to produce energy. A study published in *Clinical Nutrition* found that carnitine supplementation can improve insulin sensitivity and reduce markers of inflammation, particularly in individuals with metabolic syndrome. By enhancing fatty acid oxidation, carnitine not only supports energy production but also helps reduce the accumulation of lipid intermediates that can contribute to inflammation and insulin resistance. However, carnitine should be taken on a short-term basis for oral intake, particularly until the gut biome is better understood, as it can increase the conversion of trimethylamine (TMA) to trimethylamine N-oxide (TMAO), which may raise the risk of heart disease. Imagine carnitine as a transport vehicle that delivers fuel directly to the mitochondria, enabling efficient energy production while minimizing the toxic buildup that can harm cellular health.

Berberine is a bioactive compound found in several plants, including goldenseal and barberry. It has demonstrated potent anti-inflammatory and insulin-sensitizing effects. Research published in *Metabolism* shows that berberine can significantly lower blood sugar levels and improve metabolic health by activating AMP-activated protein kinase (AMPK), a critical enzyme that regulates energy metabolism. AMPK activation leads to improved glucose uptake and enhanced mitochondrial function, reducing oxidative stress and inflammation. Berberine also modulates gut microbiota, contributing to its anti-inflammatory effects and promoting a healthier gut environment, which is essential for maintaining cellular health. Think of berberine as a dual-action agent that not only helps lower blood sugar but also addresses the root causes of inflammation.

Alpha Lipoic Acid

Alpha-lipoic acid (ALA) is a powerful antioxidant that helps combat oxidative stress and inflammation at the cellular level. According to research in *Diabetes Care*, alpha-lipoic acid supplementation can improve insulin sensitivity and reduce symptoms associated with diabetic neuropathy. ALA is unique in that it is both water- and fat-soluble, allowing it to act in various cellular compartments. It scavenges free radicals and regenerates other antioxidants, protecting mitochondria from oxidative damage. By reducing oxidative stress, ALA helps improve mitochondrial function, which is crucial for energy production and overall cellular health. Picture ALA as a protective shield that safeguards cells from oxidative harm, ensuring they function optimally.

Curcumin

The active compound in turmeric, curcumin, is renowned for its anti-inflammatory properties. Studies have shown that curcumin can inhibit the activation of nuclear factor kappa B (NF-κB), a key regulator of inflammation. By modulating inflammatory pathways, curcumin helps alleviate chronic inflammation and improve insulin sensitivity. Research indicates that curcumin supplementation reduces inflammation markers and supports metabolic health, making it a valuable addition to any regimen aimed at combating chronic inflammation and insulin resistance.

Omega-3 Fatty Acids

Found in fish oil and flaxseed oil, omega-3 fatty acids have been extensively studied for their anti-inflammatory effects. They can lower levels of pro-inflammatory cytokines and enhance insulin sensitivity, making them a valuable addition to the diet for individuals struggling with chronic inflammation and insulin resistance.

Vitamin D

Vitamin D is an essential nutrient that plays a significant role in immune function and inflammation regulation. Research shows that adequate vitamin D levels are associated with improved insulin sensitivity and reduced markers of inflammation. Ensuring sufficient vitamin D intake through sunlight exposure or supplementation may help mitigate the effects of chronic inflammation and support overall health.

By incorporating these supplements into a comprehensive approach that includes dietary and lifestyle changes, individuals can effectively address chronic inflammation and insulin resistance, enhancing their overall health and well-being. It is important to consult with a healthcare professional before starting any new supplement regimen, as they can provide personalized advice based on individual health needs and conditions.

The combined effects of proper nutrition, regular physical activity, adequate sleep, stress management, and targeted supplementation can create a synergistic approach to improving cellular health, reducing the risk of chronic diseases, and promoting a more vibrant life.

Conclusion

Chronic inflammation and insulin resistance are two of the most significant threats to cellular health. By understanding the mechanisms behind these conditions and recognizing their symptoms, individuals can take proactive steps to improve their health. Implementing dietary and lifestyle strategies, engaging in regular physical activity, prioritizing sleep, managing stress, and considering appropriate supplements can significantly reduce inflammation, enhance insulin sensitivity, and support mitochondrial function. Taking these proactive steps not only protects against chronic disease but also promotes long-term vitality and cellular resilience.

In the next chapter, we will explore hydration and its critical role in cellular function, examining how proper hydration supports cellular health and vitality.

CHAPTER FIVE

Hydration and Cellular Function

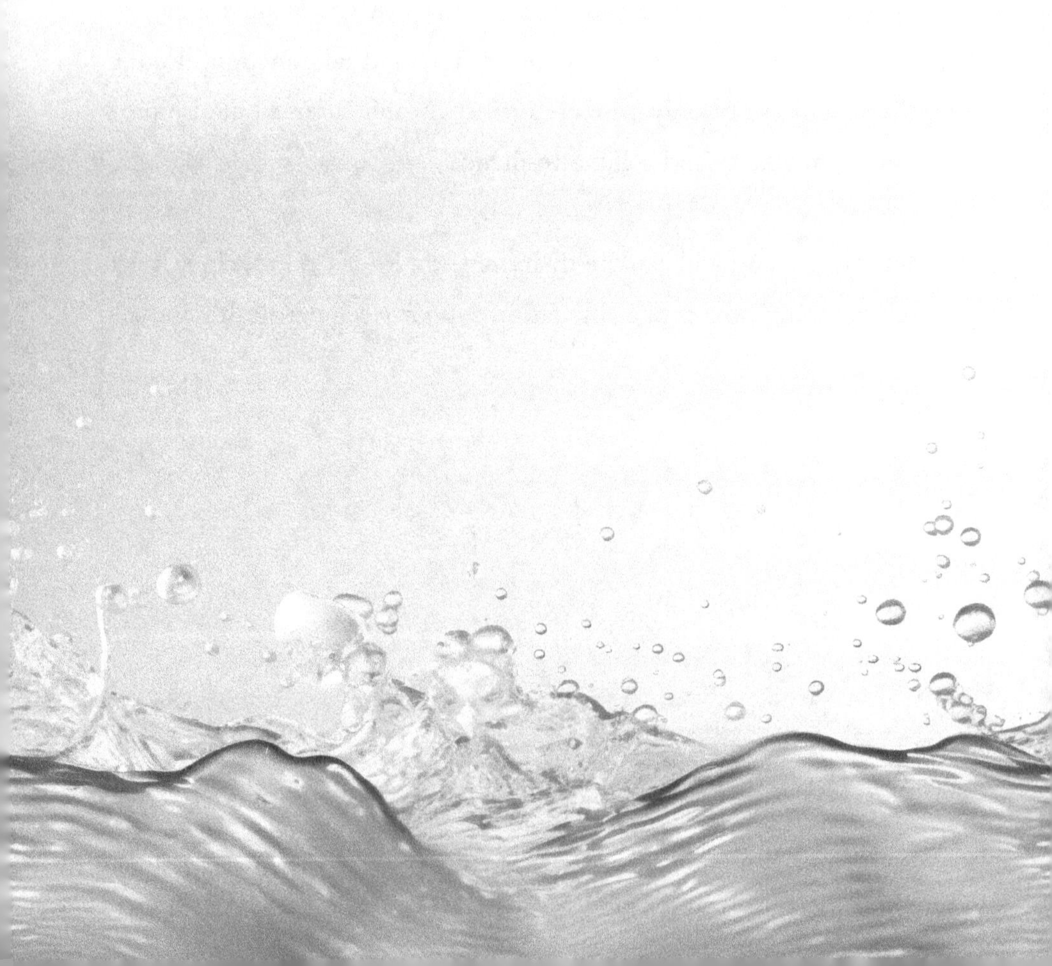

Leonardo da Vinci's profound statement, "Water is the driving force of all nature," underscores the vital role water plays in sustaining life. Just as nature depends on water to nourish ecosystems, the human body relies on proper hydration to maintain cellular function. Every cell requires water to perform essential tasks, including energy production, nutrient transport, detoxification, and waste removal. In this chapter, we explore the critical importance of hydration for cellular health, strategies to optimize hydration, and how water supports the body's detoxification processes.

The Importance of Hydration for Optimal Cellular Function

Water is essential for life and plays a key role in maintaining the structure and function of cells. Approximately 60% of the human body is composed of water, and every physiological process depends on adequate hydration to function properly. Water acts not only as a medium for transporting nutrients and removing waste but also as a key player in the chemical reactions that produce energy within cells.

At the cellular level, water is crucial for maintaining the balance of electrolytes—charged minerals that help regulate various physiological processes. Sodium (Na^+) and potassium (K^+) ions are vital for generating electrical impulses in neurons and muscle cells, processes necessary for communication and contraction. The movement of these electrolytes across cell membranes occurs through osmosis and diffusion, both of which depend on proper hydration. Without adequate water, the balance of electrolytes can be disrupted, leading to conditions like muscle cramps, arrhythmias, or cognitive deficits.

Water also plays a significant role in thermoregulation, the process of maintaining an optimal body temperature. As the body generates heat during physical activity, water absorbs excess heat, and through sweating, helps cool the body down. This is crucial because high temperatures can denature proteins—altering their structure and function, which can severely disrupt cellular processes. Proper hydration, therefore, acts like a coolant in an engine, preventing overheating and ensuring that cellular machinery operates smoothly.

According to a study published in *The American Journal of Physiology*, even mild dehydration can impair cellular function by reducing energy production, nutrient absorption, and detoxification efficiency. When cells lack sufficient water, they struggle to maintain homeostasis—the delicate balance necessary for optimal functioning. This struggle can manifest in a range of health issues, from fatigue and cognitive decline (often referred to as "brain fog") to compromised immune responses and increased susceptibility to illness.

One of the most critical roles of water in the body is its ability to maintain the fluidity of the cell membrane. The membrane, primarily composed of a lipid bilayer, requires adequate hydration to maintain its flexibility and permeability. This fluidity is vital for the proper functioning of membrane proteins involved in transport and signaling. When dehydration occurs, the lipid bilayer becomes rigid, impairing its ability to transport nutrients into the cell and expel waste products.

Cellular Energy

The relationship between hydration and cellular energy production cannot be overstated. Water is not just a bystander in the biochemical reactions that occur in the mitochondria; it is an active participant. For example, during glycolysis—the first step of glucose metabolism—water molecules assist in breaking down glucose into pyruvate, preparing it for entry into the mitochondria. Once inside, hydration is vital for the Krebs cycle (citric acid cycle) and the electron transport chain, both of which are responsible for the majority of ATP production. Here, water molecules help transport electrons through the chain and regulate the enzymatic activity necessary for ATP synthesis.

In a state of dehydration, the efficiency of these processes can be significantly impaired. The mitochondria may struggle to produce ATP due to the lack of water necessary for these biochemical reactions. This inefficiency can lead to a cascading effect, where reduced ATP levels cause cellular dysfunction, decreased metabolic rate, and ultimately fatigue. Individuals may feel lethargic or mentally foggy—similar to trying to drive a car with a low fuel tank. Without enough energy, the system eventually stalls.

Cell Membrane Health

Water is vital for maintaining the integrity and functionality of cell membranes. The lipid bilayer of the cell membrane requires hydration to stay flexible. Proper hydration allows phospholipids to move freely, facilitating effective signaling, nutrient transport, and waste removal. When dehydration occurs, the membrane becomes rigid and less permeable, impairing the cell's ability to take in essential nutrients and expel waste products.

On a physiological level, dehydration leads to increased intracellular calcium levels, which can trigger apoptosis (programmed cell death) and cellular senescence (a state in which cells lose their ability to divide and function effectively). This cellular senescence contributes to tissue aging and the development of chronic diseases. It's similar to a poorly maintained fence that begins to lean and rot; eventually, it fails to protect the garden it was meant to enclose, leading to further deterioration of the plants within. When cell membranes are compromised, cells lose their ability to communicate effectively, triggering stress that can provoke inflammatory responses harmful to overall health.

Cellular Terrain Health

Hydration also plays a crucial role in maintaining the cellular terrain—the extracellular matrix (ECM) surrounding cells. The ECM provides structural support, regulates nutrient flow, and facilitates communication between cells. Water acts as both a lubricant and a medium for transporting nutrients and waste products, ensuring that the ECM remains hydrated and functional.

When dehydration occurs, the ECM becomes less effective at supporting cellular functions, leading to nutrient deficiencies and an accumulation of waste products. This creates a hostile environment for cells, fostering chronic inflammation and impairing cellular repair mechanisms. A well-hydrated ECM ensures that nutrients diffuse readily to cells while waste products are efficiently removed. When the body is dehydrated, the ECM can thicken, impeding nutrient and waste transport, which further exacerbates cellular dysfunction.

The importance of hydration for maintaining the ECM's integrity cannot be overstated. Water helps maintain the viscosity of the ECM, enabling the movement of nutrients, growth factors, and hormones essential for cellular health. Think of hydration as the necessary moisture in a sponge; without it, the sponge becomes dry and rigid, unable to absorb or release effectively. Similarly, dehydration can lead to an inefficient ECM that hampers cellular communication and nutrient delivery, ultimately compromising health.

Hydration and Detoxification: Water's Role in Flushing Toxins from the Body

Hydration is not only essential for cellular function but also plays a critical role in the body's detoxification processes. Water helps flush toxins, metabolic waste products, and harmful substances out of the body, supporting the health of the kidneys, liver, and lymphatic system.

The kidneys are the body's primary filtration organs, responsible for removing waste products and excess substances from the bloodstream. They rely on adequate water intake to filter out toxins and maintain a proper balance of electrolytes. According to a study published in *Kidney International,* when the body is dehydrated, the kidneys cannot function optimally, leading to the buildup of waste products in the bloodstream. Drinking enough water helps the kidneys filter blood efficiently, producing urine that carries toxins out of the body. Proper hydration also reduces the risk of kidney stones, which can form when minerals and waste products crystallize in the kidneys due to concentrated urine.

The liver is another vital organ involved in detoxification. It processes and breaks down toxins, drugs, and other harmful substances, converting them into compounds that can be excreted from the body. According to research published in *The Journal of Hepatology*, proper hydration supports liver function by ensuring that toxins can be processed and eliminated efficiently. When the body is dehydrated, the liver's ability to detoxify is impaired, leading to the accumulation of toxins that can harm cellular health. Drinking water supports the liver in flushing out these toxins and maintaining overall cellular function.

The lymphatic system is responsible for transporting waste products, toxins, and excess fluids from the tissues and cells back into the bloodstream, where they can be eliminated. Water is essential for maintaining the flow of lymph fluid, which helps remove toxins and supports immune function. According to a study in *Lymphatic Research and Biology*, dehydration can slow down lymphatic circulation, leading to the accumulation of toxins and waste products in the tissues. Staying properly hydrated ensures that the lymphatic system can effectively remove waste and support the immune system in protecting the body from infections.

The skin, one of the body's largest organs, also plays a role in detoxification through sweating. Sweating helps release toxins, such as heavy metals and environmental pollutants, from the body. According to The Journal of Environmental and Public Health, regular hydration supports skin health by promoting sweat production, which aids in the elimination of toxins.

Proper hydration also helps maintain the skin's elasticity and prevents dryness, which can impair its ability to act as a barrier against pathogens and environmental stressors. Drinking enough water, along with practices like sauna use or exercise, can enhance sweating and support the body's natural detoxification processes.

Water is also key to digestion and helps flush toxins through the gastrointestinal system. Adequate hydration ensures that waste is effectively moved through the intestines, reducing the risk of constipation and promoting regular bowel movements. According to a study published in *The American Journal of Gastroenterology*, proper hydration helps prevent the buildup of toxins in the digestive tract and supports the liver's detoxification processes. Drinking water before and during meals aids in digestion by helping break down food, allowing nutrients to be absorbed more efficiently. This supports cellular function by ensuring that cells receive the nutrients they need for energy production, repair, and detoxification.

Signs and Symptoms of Dehydration

Dehydration can manifest in various ways, and recognizing these signs is crucial for maintaining optimal cellular health. On a cellular level, even mild dehydration can lead to symptoms such as fatigue, dizziness, confusion, and impaired cognitive function. This is because water is essential for maintaining blood flow and nutrient delivery; when hydration is lacking, the body prioritizes vital functions over cellular health, leading to a cascade of issues.

Individuals may also experience physical symptoms like dry mouth, thirst, dark yellow urine, headaches, and decreased urine output. The implications of dehydration extend beyond immediate discomfort; chronic dehydration can contribute to long-term health issues, such as kidney stones, urinary tract infections, and hypertension. In severe cases, it may lead to acute kidney injury, where the kidneys are unable to filter blood effectively due to a lack of fluid. This can create a dangerous cycle, as the accumulation of toxins from impaired kidney function further stresses the cells, leading to cellular damage and dysfunction.

Hydration Strategies: How Water, Electrolytes, and Minerals Support Cellular Health

Maintaining proper hydration involves more than just drinking water. Electrolytes and minerals are also vital for ensuring cells can maintain their internal environment and function efficiently.

Drinking enough water is essential for staying hydrated. The amount of water a person needs varies based on factors like age, activity level, climate, and overall health. A general guideline is to consume 8-10 cups (64-80 ounces) of water per day, though individual needs may differ. According to a study published in *The Journal of Clinical Endocrinology & Metabolism*, drinking water throughout the day helps the body regulate temperature, maintain blood volume, and transport nutrients.

Electrolytes are minerals with an electric charge that help maintain fluid balance inside and outside of cells. Key electrolytes include sodium, potassium, magnesium, and calcium. These minerals regulate the movement of water between cells and the extracellular space, ensuring cells stay properly hydrated. Foods rich in electrolytes—such as bananas (potassium), leafy greens (magnesium), dairy products (calcium), and moderate amounts of salty foods (sodium)—can help maintain electrolyte balance and support hydration.

In addition to drinking water, consuming water-rich foods can help maintain hydration and provide essential nutrients. Many fruits and vegetables are high in water content and contribute to overall hydration. For instance, cucumbers, watermelon, oranges, strawberries, and lettuce are composed of more than 90% water. These foods not only hydrate the body but also deliver important vitamins, minerals, and antioxidants that support cellular health.

Herbal teas and other natural beverages can also contribute to hydration while offering additional health benefits. Green tea, for example, contains antioxidants that help neutralize free radicals and reduce inflammation, promoting cellular health. Coconut water is another excellent source of hydration, as it is rich in electrolytes like potassium and magnesium. It's important to avoid sugary, caffeinated, and alcohol-based beverages, as these can dehydrate the body by increasing urine output and impairing its ability to retain water.

You can monitor your hydration levels by checking the color of your urine. Clear or pale yellow urine typically indicates good hydration, while darker yellow or amber-colored urine may suggest dehydration. Paying attention to these signs can help ensure that hydration levels are maintained. According to research published in *The American Journal of Clinical Nutrition*, individuals who track their water intake and adjust hydration based on environmental factors and activity levels are better able to maintain optimal cellular function and performance.

Conclusion

Hydration is essential for maintaining optimal cellular function and supporting the body's detoxification processes. Water is not merely a passive element; it plays an active role in every cellular process, from energy production to nutrient transport and waste removal. By consuming adequate water, electrolytes, and hydrating foods, we can ensure that our cells function efficiently and are protected from damage caused by toxins and dehydration. Whether supporting the kidneys, liver, or lymphatic system, water plays a crucial role in flushing out waste and maintaining a clean cellular environment, promoting overall health and vitality.

In the next chapter, we will explore the relationship between sunlight and energy, examining how exposure to sunlight influences cellular health, energy production, and overall vitality.

CHAPTER SIX

Sunlight and Energy

Helen Keller's quote, "Keep your face to the sun and you will never see the shadows," speaks not only to the power of a positive mindset but also to the vital role of sunlight in our lives. Sunlight has been a source of life and energy for millennia, playing a crucial role in the growth of plants, the regulation of human circadian rhythms, and the synthesis of essential nutrients in the body. As an indispensable element of our health and well-being, sunlight has the power to boost cellular function, enhance energy levels, and support immune health. In this chapter, we will explore how sunlight impacts mitochondrial function, the synthesis of vitamin D, the effects of sunlight deficiency, and the use of red light and near-infrared therapy to enhance cellular health.

The Role of Sunlight in Boosting Mitochondrial Function and Cellular Energy

Sunlight is the most abundant and accessible source of energy on Earth. For humans, exposure to sunlight triggers a series of biological processes essential for maintaining optimal health. Sunlight regulates our sleep-wake cycles, boosts mood, supports hormone production, and, importantly, plays a key role in energy production at the cellular level. The sun's rays, particularly ultraviolet (UV) light, penetrate the skin and stimulate the production of vitamin D, a crucial hormone that regulates immune function, bone health, and calcium metabolism.

Beyond vitamin D, sunlight exposure also activates mitochondrial function, enhancing the ability of cells to produce adenosine triphosphate (ATP), the molecule that powers nearly every cellular process. According to a study published in *Photochemical & Photobiological Sciences*, exposure to sunlight, especially red and near-infrared light, enhances mitochondrial function by increasing the activity of cytochrome c oxidase, an enzyme in the electron transport chain responsible for ATP production. By stimulating mitochondria to produce more ATP, sunlight increases energy levels, supports cellular repair, and enhances overall vitality.

Mitochondria are the powerhouses of the cell, responsible for converting the energy from food into ATP. When mitochondria function optimally, they produce energy efficiently, allowing cells to carry out vital tasks such as detoxification, repair, and immune defense. Sunlight exposure boosts mitochondrial function by increasing ATP production, reducing oxidative stress, and promoting cellular health.

The benefits of sunlight on mitochondrial function go beyond ATP production. Sunlight also triggers the release of endorphins, hormones that improve mood and reduce stress, which further supports cellular health by reducing inflammation and oxidative damage. Additionally, sunlight exposure helps regulate circadian rhythms, ensuring that cells have the energy they need during the day and can repair themselves at night. In sum, sunlight is a powerful natural tool for enhancing mitochondrial function and cellular energy. Regular exposure can improve physical performance, increase mental clarity, and support long-term health and longevity by optimizing cellular processes.

Vitamin D and Cellular Health: The Impact of Sunlight on Vitamin D Synthesis and Its Importance for the Immune System

Vitamin D, often called the "sunshine vitamin," is synthesized in the body when the skin is exposed to ultraviolet B (UVB) rays from the sun. It is a vital nutrient for bone health and a critical regulator of the immune system, inflammation, and overall cellular function. Without adequate sunlight exposure, the body's ability to produce vitamin D diminishes, leading to a variety of health problems, including weakened immune function, increased susceptibility to infections, and chronic inflammation.

Synthesis of Vitamin D

When the skin is exposed to UVB rays, a form of cholesterol called 7-dehydrocholesterol is converted into vitamin D3 (cholecalciferol). This inactive form of vitamin D is then transported to the liver and kidneys, where it is converted into its active form, calcitriol. Calcitriol functions as a hormone, regulating calcium and phosphate levels in the blood and ensuring proper bone mineralization. According to a study in *The Journal of Endocrinology*, vitamin D also plays a critical role in regulating immune responses. Calcitriol binds to vitamin D receptors (VDRs) on immune cells—such as macrophages, dendritic cells, and T cells—modulating their activity and reducing the risk of chronic inflammation and autoimmune diseases.

The Role of Vitamin D in Immune Health

Vitamin D has both direct and indirect effects on the immune system. Directly, it enhances the pathogen-fighting capabilities of monocytes and macrophages, key components of the innate immune system. It also supports the production of antimicrobial peptides, which help the body combat infections. Indirectly, vitamin D modulates the adaptive immune response by regulating the activity of T cells and B cells, which are responsible for targeting specific pathogens.

According to research published in *Nature Reviews Immunology*, vitamin D deficiency is associated with an increased risk of autoimmune diseases, such as multiple sclerosis, rheumatoid arthritis, and type 1 diabetes, as well as a higher susceptibility to respiratory infections. Adequate vitamin D levels help balance the immune system, reducing the risk of overactive immune responses that can lead to chronic inflammation. By enhancing the body's ability to fight infections and modulating inflammatory processes, vitamin D supports cellular health and reduces the risk of chronic diseases.

Vitamin D and Inflammation

Chronic inflammation is a major contributor to a wide range of health issues, including heart disease, diabetes, and neurodegenerative disorders. Vitamin D plays an anti-inflammatory role by inhibiting the production of pro-inflammatory cytokines and promoting the production of anti-inflammatory cytokines. This balance helps prevent excessive inflammation that can damage tissues and impair cellular function. According to a study in *The Journal of Clinical Endocrinology & Metabolism*, individuals with low vitamin D levels have higher levels of inflammatory markers, such as C-reactive protein (CRP) and tumor necrosis factor-alpha (TNF-α). Increasing vitamin D levels through sunlight exposure or supplementation can reduce inflammation, supporting overall health and protecting against chronic disease.

In addition to its role in immune regulation and inflammation, vitamin D supports mitochondrial function by promoting calcium homeostasis and reducing oxidative stress. Calcium is essential for ATP production in the mitochondria, and vitamin D helps regulate calcium levels in both the blood and cells. Furthermore, vitamin D's antioxidant properties protect mitochondria from oxidative damage caused by free radicals. According to a study in *The Journal of Biological Chemistry*, vitamin D deficiency is associated with mitochondrial dysfunction, reduced ATP production, and increased oxidative stress. Ensuring adequate vitamin D levels through sunlight exposure supports mitochondrial health, enhances energy production, and protects cells from oxidative damage.

Sunlight and Light Therapies for Enhanced Cellular Health

Sunlight is a powerful natural source of energy that plays a critical role in boosting mitochondrial function, enhancing cellular repair, and supporting immune health. By stimulating the production of vitamin D, sunlight strengthens the immune system, reduces inflammation, and protects against chronic diseases. In addition to natural sunlight, specific light frequencies—such as red and near-infrared light—offer significant health benefits by further enhancing mitochondrial function, promoting cellular repair, and reducing inflammation. Incorporating regular sunlight exposure and light therapies into daily routines can improve energy levels, support recovery from injury, and enhance overall health and well-being. Whether through natural sunlight or therapeutic light devices, harnessing the power of light is an effective strategy for optimizing cellular health, promoting longevity, and reducing the risk of chronic disease.

Signs and Symptoms of Sunlight Deficiency

A deficiency in sunlight exposure can manifest in various ways, impacting both physical and mental health. One of the most common signs of insufficient sunlight is low levels of vitamin D, which can lead to symptoms such as fatigue, muscle weakness, and bone pain. This deficiency can also contribute to mood disorders, including seasonal affective disorder (SAD), characterized by depression during the winter months when sunlight exposure is limited. The impact of low vitamin D levels on immune function can increase susceptibility to infections and chronic diseases.

Another indicator of sunlight deficiency is increased chronic inflammation. Lower levels of vitamin D can elevate inflammatory markers in the body, creating a vicious cycle where chronic inflammation further suppresses the immune system and reduces the body's ability to respond effectively to pathogens.

Red Light and Near-Infrared Therapy: How Specific Light Frequencies Enhance Cellular Health

Similar to natural sunlight, specific light frequencies—such as red light and near-infrared light—have been shown to offer significant health benefits by enhancing mitochondrial function, reducing inflammation, and promoting cellular repair. Red light and near-infrared therapy are emerging as powerful tools for improving cellular health, particularly for individuals with chronic conditions, injuries, or fatigue.

The Science Behind Red Light and Near-Infrared Therapy

Red light (600–700 nm) and near-infrared light (700–1200 nm) are forms of low-level light therapy (LLLT) that penetrate the skin and are absorbed by the mitochondria. These wavelengths of light stimulate the activity of cytochrome c oxidase, an enzyme in the electron transport chain that plays a critical role in ATP production. According to a study published in *Photomedicine and Laser Surgery*, red and near-infrared light therapy increases mitochondrial function by enhancing ATP production, reducing oxidative stress, and improving cellular energy metabolism. By stimulating mitochondrial activity, red light therapy helps cells generate more energy, repair damage, and function more efficiently.

Red Light Therapy and Cellular Repair

Red light therapy is particularly effective at promoting cellular repair and regeneration, making it a valuable tool for healing wounds, reducing inflammation, and supporting recovery from injuries. According to a study in *Lasers in Surgery and Medicine*, red light therapy enhances collagen production, a protein essential for tissue repair and skin health. By stimulating collagen synthesis and reducing inflammation, red light therapy accelerates wound healing, minimizes scarring, and supports tissue regeneration. This therapy is also widely used in dermatology to treat conditions like acne, psoriasis, and eczema, as it reduces inflammation and promotes healthy skin cell turnover.

Near-Infrared Therapy and Muscle Recovery

Near-infrared therapy is commonly used to enhance muscle recovery and reduce pain and inflammation following intense physical activity. Research published in *The Journal of Athletic Training* indicates that near-infrared light penetrates deeper into tissues than red light, making it particularly effective for treating muscle soreness, joint pain, and inflammation. Near-infrared therapy enhances blood flow to the muscles, delivering oxygen and nutrients while helping to clear metabolic waste products that contribute to soreness and inflammation. By improving circulation and reducing oxidative stress, near-infrared therapy aids in faster recovery and reduces the risk of injury.

The Anti-Inflammatory Effects of Red and Near-Infrared Light

One of the most significant benefits of red and near-infrared light therapy is its ability to reduce inflammation at the cellular level. While inflammation is a natural response to injury or infection, chronic inflammation can lead to tissue damage and contribute to conditions like arthritis, heart disease, and neurodegenerative disorders. According to a study published in *The Journal of Photochemistry and Photobiology*, red and near-infrared light therapy reduces the production of pro-inflammatory cytokines and boosts the production of anti-inflammatory cytokines. This helps balance the immune response, reducing the risk of chronic inflammation that can damage tissues and impair cellular function.

Recent research has explored the potential of red and near-infrared light therapy to enhance cognitive function and protect against neurodegenerative diseases like Alzheimer's and Parkinson's. A study in *Neurobiology of Aging* found that near-infrared light therapy improves mitochondrial function in brain cells, reduces oxidative stress, and enhances cognitive performance. Both red and near-infrared light therapy have been shown to promote neurogenesis (the growth of new neurons) and improve blood flow to the brain, both of which are essential for maintaining cognitive function and preventing neurodegenerative diseases. These therapies may also help reduce the accumulation of amyloid plaques, which are associated with Alzheimer's disease.

Suggested Plan for Sun Exposure

To maximize the health benefits of sunlight, aim for 15-20 minutes of sun exposure daily, preferably during the morning or late afternoon when UV radiation is less intense. Here are some tips for safe sun exposure:

- **Choose the Right Time**: Aim for exposure between 10 a.m. and 3 p.m., when UVB rays are most effective for vitamin D synthesis. Be mindful of your skin type and local UV index.
- **Start Slowly**: If you have sensitive skin or are not used to sun exposure, start with shorter durations and gradually increase the time spent in the sun.

- **Protect Your Skin**: After 15-20 minutes of sun exposure, apply a non-toxic sunscreen with broad-spectrum protection to prevent skin damage, especially if you plan to stay outside longer.
- **Consider Dietary Support**: Ensure your diet includes foods rich in healthy fats, such as avocados, nuts, and fish, which help with the absorption of vitamin D.
- **Supplement Wisely**: If natural sunlight is not accessible, consider supplementing with vitamin D3 and K2 to enhance absorption and prevent calcium misplacement in the body.
- **Alternative Therapies**: If sunlight exposure is limited due to geographic location or lifestyle, consider using photobiomodulation or red-light therapy devices to mimic sunlight's benefits on cellular health and mitochondrial function.

Conclusion

Incorporating sunlight exposure into our daily routines is essential for enhancing cellular function, optimizing energy levels, and supporting overall health. By understanding the biochemical processes behind sunlight, vitamin D synthesis, and the benefits of red-light therapy, we can harness the power of light to promote cellular vitality. Protecting our skin with non-toxic sunscreens, monitoring vitamin D levels, and considering alternative therapies when sunlight is scarce will help ensure we reap the full benefits of this natural resource.

In the next chapter, we will explore the vital connection between sleep and cellular restoration, uncovering how proper sleep hygiene is crucial for maintaining cellular health and ensuring optimal functioning of our bodies.

CHAPTER SEVEN

Sleep and Cellular Restoration

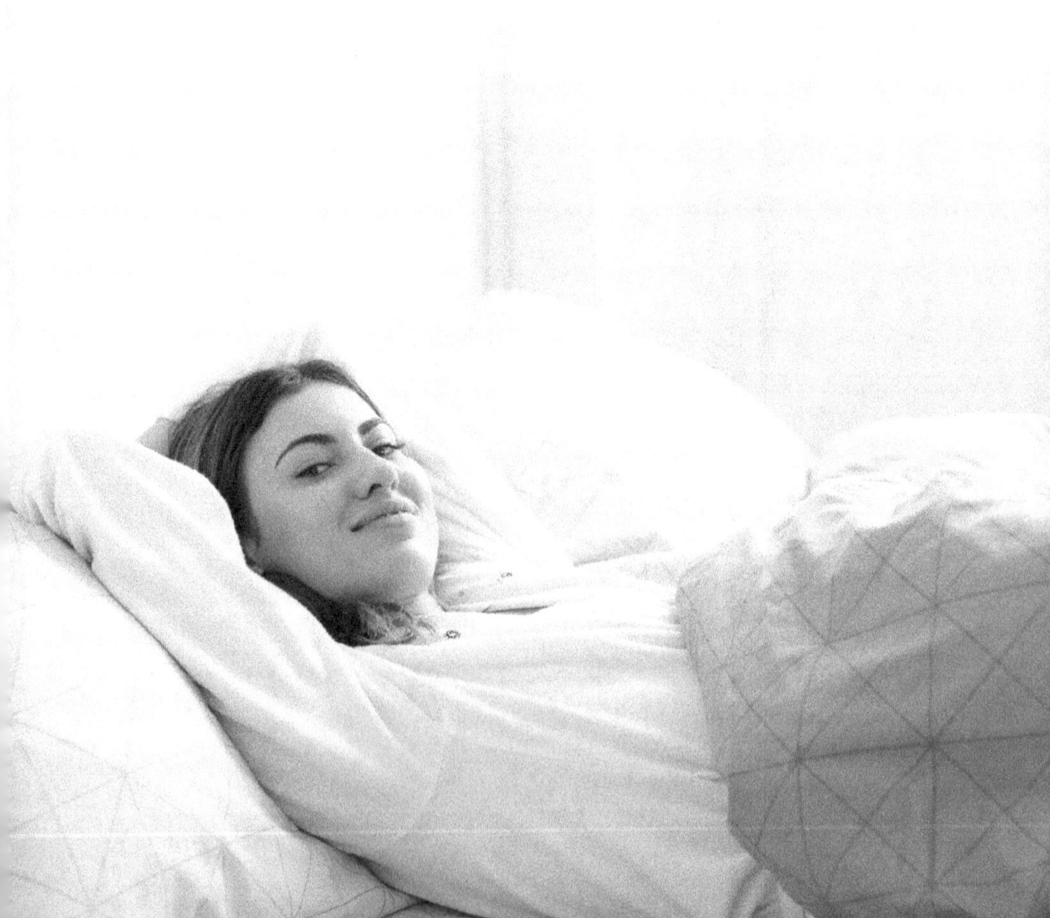

"Sleep is the best meditation." —*Dalai Lama*

The Dalai Lama's profound words, "Sleep is the best meditation," underscore the essential role of sleep in restoring both body and mind. Sleep is a natural, regenerative state critical for health and well-being. During sleep, the body undergoes complex processes that allow cells to repair, regenerate, and detoxify. It is through sleep that the brain processes emotions, the immune system strengthens, and damaged tissues are repaired. This chapter explores the vital connection between sleep and cellular health, focusing on the physiological processes that occur during rest, the importance of melatonin as a cellular protector, and practical strategies for optimizing sleep to enhance cellular function and overall healing.

The Role of Sleep in Repairing and Regenerating Cells

Sleep is often viewed as a period of rest for the body and mind, but in reality, it is a highly active state of restoration and healing. During sleep, the body shifts into repair mode, performing essential functions such as cellular regeneration, detoxification, and immune strengthening. The sleep process is divided into several stages, including light sleep, deep sleep, and rapid eye movement (REM) sleep. Each of these stages plays a unique role in maintaining cellular health and promoting overall vitality.

According to research in Nature Reviews Neuroscience, sleep is essential for the proper functioning of every system in the body, including the immune, cardiovascular, and nervous systems. Sleep allows the body to perform critical repair functions that cannot occur during wakefulness, including the removal of toxins from cells, the repair of damaged DNA, and the production of proteins necessary for cellular growth and recovery. One of the most important processes that occur during sleep is autophagy, a form of cellular housekeeping that involves the breakdown and recycling of damaged or unnecessary cellular components. This process is vital for maintaining cellular health and preventing the accumulation of harmful substances that can lead to chronic diseases, such as cancer and neurodegenerative conditions.

Sleep also supports the function of the lymphatic system, which removes waste products and toxins from the brain and body. During deep sleep, the brain's glymphatic system becomes more active, flushing out toxins like beta-amyloid, a protein linked to Alzheimer's disease. According to a study published in *Science*, the brain's ability to detoxify itself during sleep is critical for preventing cognitive decline and maintaining overall brain health. In addition to its detoxification and repair functions, sleep is essential for balancing hormones that regulate hunger, stress, and energy.

Effects of Improper Sleep on Cellular Health

Improper sleep—whether insufficient, poor quality, or disrupted—has profound adverse effects on cellular health. At the cellular level, sleep deprivation disrupts critical processes, leading to a range of negative outcomes. Studies have shown that inadequate sleep leads to increased oxidative stress, which results in cellular damage. Cells rely on sleep to perform autophagy, cleaning out damaged cellular components. When this process is impaired, damaged proteins and organelles accumulate, leading to cellular dysfunction and increasing the risk of chronic diseases.

Moreover, lack of sleep elevates cortisol levels, the body's primary stress hormone. Chronically elevated cortisol can trigger inflammation by stimulating the release of pro-inflammatory cytokines, such as interleukin-6 (IL-6) and tumor necrosis factor-alpha (TNF-α). This inflammatory response contributes to a host of health issues, including metabolic syndrome, cardiovascular disease, and neurodegenerative disorders. On a physiological level, inflammation can hinder insulin signaling pathways, exacerbating insulin resistance—a condition where cells become less responsive to insulin, impairing glucose uptake and leading to elevated blood sugar levels.

Improper sleep also negatively impacts mitochondrial function. Mitochondria, the cell's energy powerhouses, rely on adequate sleep for optimal performance. A lack of sleep diminishes ATP production, leading to fatigue and reduced energy availability for essential cellular processes. Cells under energy stress become less efficient at detoxification and repair, contributing to an overall decline in health. This cellular fatigue can be compared to a car running on low fuel—it may struggle to accelerate or function properly until refueled.

How Sleep Supports Cellular Health: Discussion on Melatonin and Its Antioxidant Effects on Cells

One of the key mechanisms through which sleep supports cellular health is the production of melatonin, a hormone produced by the pineal gland in response to darkness. While melatonin is well-known for its role in regulating the sleep-wake cycle, its benefits extend far beyond sleep. Melatonin is a powerful antioxidant that helps protect cells from damage caused by free radicals and oxidative stress.

Melatonin is often referred to as the "sleep hormone" due to its role in promoting sleepiness and regulating the circadian rhythm—the body's internal clock that governs the sleep-wake cycle. According to research published in *The Journal of Pineal Research*, melatonin levels rise in the evening as it gets darker, signaling to the body that it's time to sleep. Melatonin helps prepare the body for sleep by lowering body temperature, reducing cortisol levels, and promoting relaxation.

Melatonin production is directly influenced by light exposure, particularly blue light from electronic devices and artificial lighting. When the eyes are exposed to light, melatonin production is suppressed, which can delay sleep onset and reduce sleep quality. This is why it is important to minimize exposure to blue light in the evening to support healthy melatonin levels and promote restful sleep.

In addition to its role in sleep regulation, melatonin is a potent antioxidant that protects cells from oxidative stress and DNA damage. Oxidative stress occurs when there is an imbalance between free radicals (unstable molecules that can damage cells) and antioxidants in the body. Free radicals are produced during normal metabolic processes but can accumulate due to factors such as poor diet, stress, pollution, and radiation. According to a study published in *The Journal of Cellular Physiology*, melatonin neutralizes free radicals and enhances the activity of other antioxidants, including glutathione, superoxide dismutase, and catalase. This antioxidant activity is critical for protecting cells from damage that can lead to premature aging, inflammation, and chronic diseases such as cancer and cardiovascular disease.

Melatonin is unique in that it can cross the blood-brain barrier, providing protection not only to cells throughout the body but also to neurons in the brain. This makes melatonin particularly important for preventing neurodegenerative diseases such as Alzheimer's and Parkinson's, which are associated with oxidative damage to brain cells.

Melatonin and Mitochondrial Health

Mitochondria, the energy-producing organelles within cells, are essential for overall cellular health. Melatonin has been shown to support mitochondrial function by reducing oxidative stress, enhancing ATP (energy) production, and preventing mitochondrial DNA damage. According to a study published in The *Journal of Pineal Research*, melatonin protects mitochondria from damage caused by free radicals, promoting cellular energy production and preventing the decline in mitochondrial function that occurs with aging.

Melatonin also supports the process of mitochondrial biogenesis—the creation of new mitochondria—which is crucial for maintaining energy levels and preventing fatigue. By protecting mitochondria and supporting their function, melatonin enhances cellular energy production and promotes overall health and vitality.

Melatonin plays an important role in regulating immune function, particularly by reducing inflammation and supporting the activity of immune cells. According to research published in *Molecular and Cellular Endocrinology*, melatonin modulates the production of pro-inflammatory cytokines, helping to reduce chronic inflammation that can damage cells and contribute to diseases such as arthritis, heart disease, and cancer.

Melatonin also enhances the activity of natural killer (NK) cells, which are part of the body's first line of defense against infections and cancer. By supporting immune function and reducing inflammation, melatonin promotes cellular health and helps protect the body from chronic diseases.

Optimizing Sleep for Healing: Natural Ways to Improve Sleep Quality for Enhanced Cellular Function

Achieving high-quality sleep is essential for allowing the body to repair and regenerate cells, detoxify itself, and maintain optimal health. However, many individuals struggle with sleep disorders, insomnia, or poor sleep habits that impair their ability to get restorative sleep. Below are several natural strategies for improving sleep quality and supporting cellular health:

One of the most effective ways to improve sleep quality is to go to bed and wake up at the same time every day, even on weekends. This helps regulate the circadian rhythm and ensures that the body knows when it is time to sleep and when it is time to wake up. According to a study published in *Sleep Medicine Reviews*, maintaining a consistent sleep schedule improves sleep efficiency, reduces the time it takes to fall asleep, and enhances overall sleep quality. Creating a regular sleep routine that includes winding-down activities such as reading, meditation, or taking a warm bath can also signal to the body that it is time to sleep.

Create a Sleep-Friendly Environment

The environment in which you sleep can significantly impact sleep quality. Creating a dark, quiet, and cool bedroom can help promote restful sleep by reducing distractions and encouraging relaxation. Research published in *The Journal of Sleep Research* highlights that exposure to light during sleep, especially blue light from electronic devices, can disrupt melatonin production and impair sleep quality.

Using blackout curtains, removing electronic devices from the bedroom, and keeping the room at a comfortable temperature (between 60-67°F) can help create an environment that supports restorative sleep. Additionally, using white noise machines or earplugs can help reduce noise disturbances and improve sleep quality.

Minimize Blue Light Exposure

Blue light emitted by electronic devices such as smartphones, tablets, and computers can suppress melatonin production and delay sleep onset. According to a study in *Chronobiology International*, exposure to blue light in the evening can disrupt the circadian rhythm and reduce sleep quality.

To minimize the impact of blue light on sleep, it's recommended to reduce screen time during the hour leading up to bedtime. Using blue light-blocking glasses or activating "night mode" on electronic devices can also help reduce blue light exposure and support melatonin production.

Stress and anxiety are major contributors to sleep disturbances and insomnia. Practicing relaxation techniques such as deep breathing, meditation, yoga, or progressive muscle relaxation can help calm the mind and body, making it easier to fall asleep and stay asleep. According to a study published in *The Journal of Alternative and Complementary Medicine*, mindfulness meditation has been shown to improve sleep quality by reducing stress and promoting relaxation. Deep breathing exercises and progressive muscle relaxation can also activate the parasympathetic nervous system, helping promote relaxation and better sleep.

Incorporate Sleep-Promoting Nutrients and Herbs

Certain nutrients and herbs can support sleep by promoting relaxation, reducing stress, and enhancing melatonin production. Some of the most effective sleep-promoting nutrients and herbs include:

- **Magnesium**: Magnesium plays a key role in regulating the nervous system and promoting relaxation. According to a study in *The Journal of Research in Medical Sciences*, magnesium supplementation has been shown to improve sleep quality, reduce insomnia, and promote relaxation.

- **L-Theanine**: L-Theanine, an amino acid found in green tea, promotes relaxation without causing drowsiness. Research published in *Nutritional Neuroscience* suggests that L-Theanine helps reduce stress, improve sleep quality, and enhance relaxation.

- **Valerian Root**: Valerian root is an herb commonly used to promote relaxation and improve sleep quality. A study in *Phytotherapy Research* found that valerian root has sedative properties, helping to reduce the time it takes to fall asleep and enhancing overall sleep quality.

- **Lavender**: Lavender is known for its calming effects and ability to reduce anxiety. According to a study in *The Journal of Sleep Medicine & Disorders*, lavender aromatherapy has been shown to improve sleep quality and alleviate symptoms of insomnia.

- **Glycine**: This amino acid has been shown to have sleep-promoting effects by improving sleep quality and reducing daytime sleepiness. Research published in *Neuroscience Letters* indicates that glycine helps lower body temperature, which is crucial for initiating sleep and promoting relaxation.

- **Inositol**: Inositol, a carbohydrate involved in cellular signaling, has a calming effect on the brain. Research shows that inositol supplementation can reduce anxiety and improve sleep quality, particularly in individuals with insomnia or anxiety disorders. It is believed to enhance neurotransmitter function, such as serotonin, which regulates mood and sleep cycles. Including inositol in the diet may promote relaxation and support healthy sleep patterns.

Incorporating these nutrients and herbs into your diet or using them as supplements can help promote relaxation, support melatonin production, and enhance overall sleep quality.

Sleep as the Foundation of Cellular Health and Well-Being

Sleep is not just a period of rest; it is a time of intense cellular activity during which the body repairs itself, regenerates tissues, detoxifies, and restores energy. Achieving high-quality sleep is essential for maintaining cellular health, preventing chronic diseases, and promoting long-term vitality. From the production of melatonin to the detoxification of the brain, sleep is foundational for cellular restoration and overall well-being.

By optimizing sleep through consistent sleep schedules, creating a sleep-friendly environment, minimizing blue light exposure, and incorporating sleep-promoting nutrients, we can enhance the body's ability to repair and regenerate itself. Ultimately, sleep is one of the most powerful tools for healing, longevity, and resilience against the challenges of modern life.

Conclusion

In conclusion, sleep is a fundamental pillar of cellular vitality. During sleep, our bodies engage in crucial restorative processes that repair cellular damage, detoxify harmful substances, and support the optimal functioning of our immune systems. The interplay between sleep, melatonin production, and mitochondrial health underscores the intricate connections between our lifestyle choices and cellular well-being.

By prioritizing sleep and adopting strategies to enhance sleep quality, we can significantly improve our overall health, resilience, and longevity.

In the next chapter, we will explore the intricate relationship between breathing and cellular restoration, examining how the power of breath influences cellular health and energy production.

CHAPTER EIGHT

The Power of Breathing

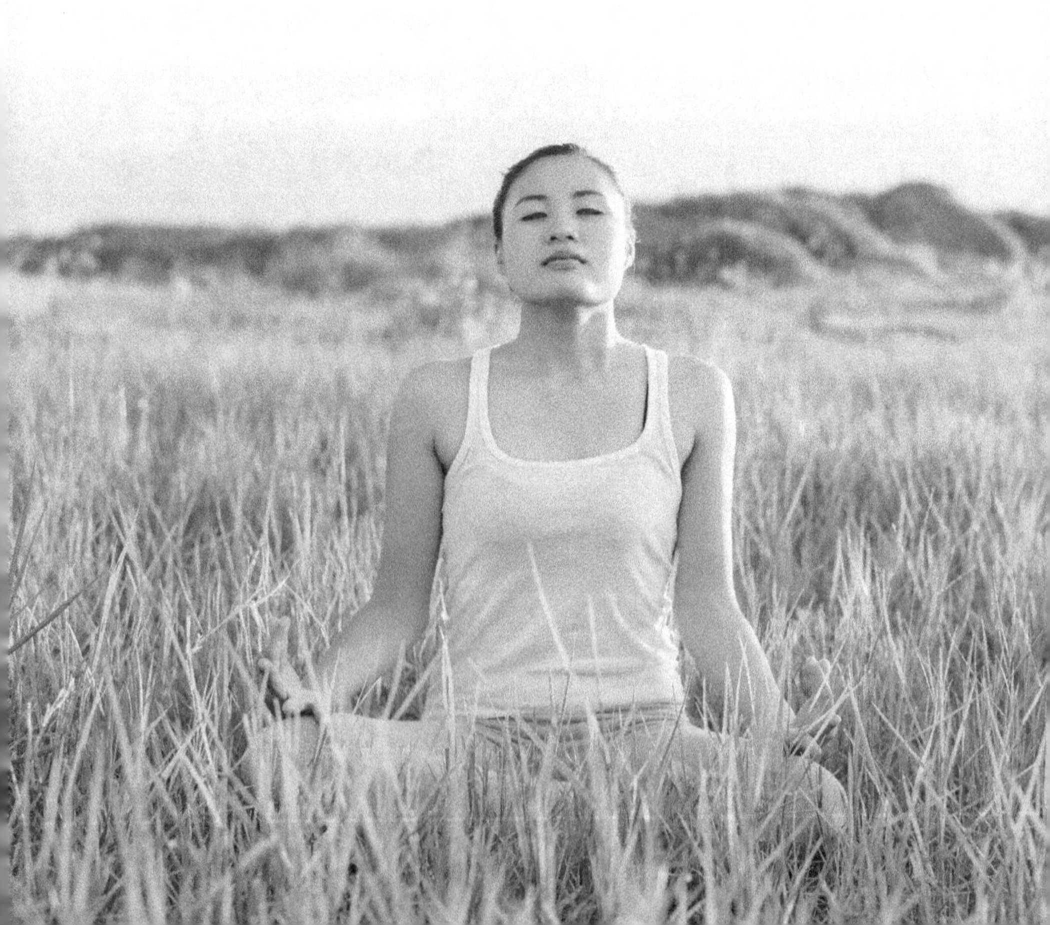

"Breath is the bridge which connects life to consciousness." —Thích Nhâ`t Hanh

Thích Nhâ`t Hanh's insightful words, "Breath is the bridge which connects life to consciousness," highlight the profound connection between breathing, life force, and awareness. Breathing is an involuntary yet fundamental act that sustains life. Every breath we take fuels cellular processes, supports mitochondrial function, and delivers oxygen to the body. Beyond sustaining life, breath is a powerful tool for healing, energy regulation, and enhancing cellular health. This chapter explores the science behind breathing, its effects on cellular energy, ancient practices like pranayama, and how proper oxygenation can promote cellular repair and vitality.

The Science Behind Breathing and Its Effect on Cellular Energy

Breathing is a critical physiological function that allows the body to take in oxygen (O_2) and expel carbon dioxide (CO_2). Oxygen is essential for producing energy at the cellular level, particularly in the mitochondria, which convert oxygen and nutrients into adenosine triphosphate (ATP)—the energy currency of the cell. Therefore, breathing is the primary mechanism through which cells receive the oxygen they need to produce energy and function optimally.

Oxygen plays a vital role in aerobic respiration, the process through which mitochondria produce ATP. During this process, oxygen acts as the final electron acceptor in the electron transport chain, facilitating ATP production while preventing the accumulation of toxic byproducts, such as free radicals. When cells don't receive enough oxygen—a condition known as hypoxia—energy production slows, and cellular function becomes impaired.

Proper breathing helps regulate blood pH levels, maintains the balance of oxygen and carbon dioxide, and supports overall homeostasis. A well-oxygenated body promotes all vital processes, from immune function to cognitive performance. Conversely, shallow or inefficient breathing can reduce oxygen delivery, increase cellular stress, and hinder cellular repair.

Modern lifestyles, characterized by high levels of stress, sedentary habits, and poor posture, often lead to shallow or dysfunctional breathing patterns. Many individuals unknowingly breathe from the chest, taking shallow breaths that don't fully engage the diaphragm—a muscle essential for deep, efficient breathing. Shallow breathing reduces the amount of oxygen available to cells, leading to fatigue, decreased mental clarity, and increased stress. According to a study published in *Respiratory Physiology & Neurobiology*, individuals who practice diaphragmatic or deep breathing experience better oxygenation, improved cellular energy production, and lower levels of stress hormones like cortisol. Breathing is not just a passive function; it is a powerful tool that can be harnessed to optimize cellular energy, enhance immune function, and promote healing. By adopting proper breathing techniques, such as deep diaphragmatic breathing or pranayama, individuals can improve oxygen delivery, boost ATP production, and support the body's natural healing processes.

Breathing Techniques for Everyone: Simple and Effective Practices

Incorporating simple breathing techniques into your daily routine can have profound effects on cellular health and overall well-being. Here are a few effective methods anyone can practice:

- Find a comfortable seated or lying position. Place one hand on your chest and the other on your abdomen.
- Inhale deeply through your nose, allowing your abdomen to rise as you fill your lungs with air. Aim for a count of four seconds.
- Hold your breath for a count of four seconds.
- Exhale slowly through your mouth, letting your abdomen fall, for a count of six seconds.
- Repeat this cycle for five to ten minutes. This practice promotes relaxation and enhances oxygen delivery to the cells.

- Inhale deeply through your nose for a count of four seconds.
- Hold your breath for a count of four seconds.
- Exhale slowly through your mouth for a count of four seconds.
- Hold your breath again for a count of four seconds.

Repeat this cycle for several minutes. Box breathing is excellent for reducing stress and anxiety, as it helps regulate the autonomic nervous system.

- Inhale quietly through your nose for a count of four seconds.
- Hold your breath for a count of seven seconds.
- Exhale completely through your mouth, making a whoosh sound, for a count of eight seconds.

- Repeat the cycle four times. This technique calms the mind and promotes deeper relaxation.

- Sit comfortably with your spine straight. Use your right thumb to close your right nostril.
- Inhale deeply through your left nostril for a count of four seconds.
- Close your left nostril with your right ring finger, open your right nostril, and exhale through the right nostril for a count of four seconds.
- Inhale through the right nostril for a count of four seconds, close the right nostril, and exhale through the left nostril for a count of four seconds.
- Continue alternating for five to ten cycles. This practice balances the body's energy and improves focus.

Pranayama and Cellular Health: Ancient Breathing Techniques to Support Mitochondrial Function

Pranayama, the ancient practice of breath control, has been used for thousands of years in yogic traditions to enhance physical, mental, and spiritual well-being. Derived from the Sanskrit words prana (life force or energy) and yama (control or regulation), pranayama encompasses a variety of breathing techniques designed to regulate the flow of prana, optimize energy levels, and promote cellular health. The physiological effects of pranayama extend far beyond relaxation and stress reduction. According to a study published in *The Journal of Alternative and Complementary Medicine*, pranayama has profound effects on the body, including enhanced oxygenation, support for mitochondrial function, and promotion of detoxification within cells.

Ujjayi Pranayama (Victorious Breath)

Ujjayi pranayama is characterized by slow, deep inhalations and exhalations through the nose, creating a soothing sound. This technique is commonly used in yoga to enhance concentration and regulate energy flow. Research published in the *International Journal of Yoga* indicates that Ujjayi pranayama improves lung capacity and increases the efficiency of oxygen exchange in the alveoli (air sacs in the lungs). Enhanced oxygenation supports mitochondrial function and ATP production, allowing cells to generate energy more efficiently. Additionally, this practice activates the parasympathetic nervous system, promoting relaxation and reducing the body's stress response. This supports cellular repair and helps reduce inflammation.

Nadi Shodhana Pranayama (Alternate Nostril Breathing)

Nadi Shodhana involves alternating the flow of breath between the left and right nostrils, which is believed to balance the brain's hemispheres and promote mental clarity. Research in *The Journal of Ayurveda and Integrative Medicine* suggests that Nadi Shodhana enhances the body's ability to absorb and utilize oxygen, promoting efficient energy production in the mitochondria. This technique reduces oxidative stress by balancing the autonomic nervous system, supporting the parasympathetic nervous response, and optimizing oxygen delivery to the brain and body.

Kapalabhati Pranayama (Skull Shining Breath)

Kapalabhati pranayama involves rapid, forceful exhalations followed by passive inhalations. Known as "skull shining breath," this technique cleanses the mind and energizes the body. According to The Journal of Human Kinetics, Kapalabhati increases oxygen uptake, improves lung function, and stimulates respiratory muscles. Enhanced oxygenation supports mitochondrial function, promotes ATP production, and boosts cellular energy levels. Kapalabhati also helps detoxify the body by stimulating the lymphatic system, aiding in the removal of metabolic waste products and toxins from the cells.

Bhramari Pranayama (Bee Breath)

Bhramari pranayama produces a humming sound during exhalation, which is known for its calming effects on the nervous system. Research in *Frontiers in Psychiatry* shows that this technique activates the parasympathetic nervous system, reducing stress hormones and promoting relaxation. By calming the mind and body, Bhramari enhances cellular repair and stimulates the vagus nerve, which regulates the immune system and helps reduce inflammation.

Sheetali Pranayama (Cooling Breath)

Sheetali pranayama involves inhaling through the mouth with a rolled tongue. This technique helps reduce heat in the body and promotes relaxation. According to a study published in *The Journal of Ayurveda and Integrative Medicine*, Sheetali pranayama can lower both body temperature and blood pressure. By reducing physiological stress, this technique supports mitochondrial function and enhances the body's ability to repair and regenerate cells.

Oxygenation and Healing: How Proper Breathing Enhances Oxygen Delivery and Promotes Cellular Repair

Oxygen is essential for life, and its role in healing and cellular repair cannot be overstated. Proper breathing ensures the body receives the oxygen it needs to fuel cellular processes, repair tissues, and support overall health. Oxygen plays a crucial role in cellular respiration, the process by which cells convert oxygen and nutrients into energy in the form of ATP. Without sufficient oxygen, cells cannot produce enough energy to function optimally, leading to fatigue, impaired healing, and increased susceptibility to illness.

Mitochondria rely on oxygen to generate ATP through oxidative phosphorylation. In this process, oxygen serves as the final electron acceptor in the electron transport chain, allowing the mitochondria to produce ATP efficiently. When oxygen levels are low, mitochondrial function is impaired, reducing ATP production and compromising cellular energy. According to research published in *Mitochondrion*, hypoxia can lead to mitochondrial dysfunction, oxidative stress, and damage to cellular structures. Proper breathing ensures that oxygen is delivered to cells in sufficient quantities, supporting mitochondrial function, enhancing energy production, and promoting cellular repair.

Oxygen is also vital for detoxifying cells and removing harmful substances. The oxidative phosphorylation process in mitochondria produces reactive oxygen species (ROS) as byproducts of cellular metabolism. While ROS play a role in cell signaling and immune responses, excessive ROS production can lead to oxidative stress, damaging DNA, proteins, and cell membranes. Proper breathing helps regulate the balance between oxygen and ROS, ensuring cells can detoxify themselves without being overwhelmed by oxidative stress. A study published in Free *Radical Biology and Medicine* suggests that deep breathing practices can enhance the body's ability to neutralize ROS and reduce oxidative damage, thereby promoting cellular health and longevity.

Breathing as a Tool for Cellular Health and Healing

Breathing is an essential yet often overlooked tool for enhancing cellular health, promoting healing, and supporting overall well-being. From ancient practices like pranayama to modern scientific research, the evidence is clear: proper breathing improves oxygen delivery, supports mitochondrial function, and promotes the body's natural ability to repair and regenerate itself. By incorporating breathing techniques into daily life, individuals can enhance oxygenation, reduce stress, and optimize cellular health. Whether through deep diaphragmatic breathing, pranayama, or simply paying attention to the breath, harnessing the power of breathing can lead to profound improvements in energy levels, mental clarity, and overall vitality. Breath is truly the bridge between life and consciousness, and by mastering it, we unlock the full potential of our cells and our health.

Conclusion

In conclusion, breathing is a powerful and essential aspect of life that direct-ly influences our cellular health and overall well-being. By understanding the physiological and biochemical roles of oxygen, the impact of breath on cellular energy production, and the benefits of practices like pranayama, we can harness the full potential of our breath. Integrating proper breathing techniques into our daily routines not only enhances oxygen delivery and energy production but also promotes relaxation, reduces stress, and supports the body's natural healing processes. As we move into Chapter 9, we will explore the concept of grounding—connecting ourselves to the Earth to further enhance cellular balance and well-being.

Grounding for Cellular Balance

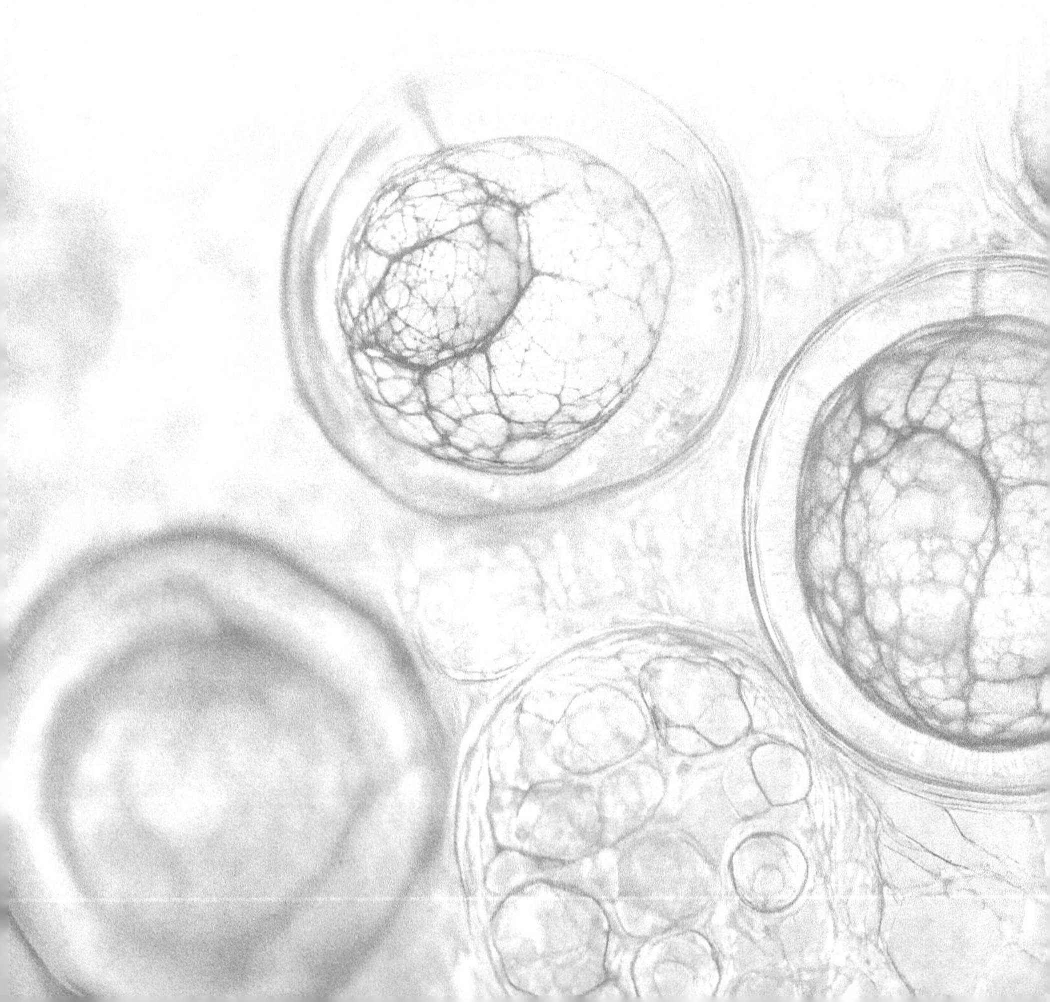

George Santayana's poetic quote, "The Earth has music for those who listen," captures the profound connection between humans and the natural world. The Earth sustains all life, providing not only the resources we need but also a subtle, often overlooked form of healing energy. Grounding, or earthing, is the practice of reconnecting with the Earth's natural energy by making direct physical contact with its surface. For centuries, people lived in closer connection with nature—walking barefoot and sleeping on the ground—but modern lifestyles have disconnected us from this primal source of balance. In recent years, scientific research has begun to uncover the health benefits of grounding, particularly its ability to reduce inflammation, improve sleep, and enhance cellular function. This chapter will explore how grounding supports cellular health, the scientific studies backing its effectiveness, and practical ways to incorporate grounding into daily life.

How Grounding (Earthing) Supports Cellular Function

Grounding is based on the idea that direct contact with the Earth's surface allows the body to absorb electrons from the ground. These electrons act as powerful antioxidants, neutralizing harmful free radicals and reducing oxidative stress, a key driver of chronic inflammation and cellular damage. According to a study published in *The Journal of Environmental and Public Health*, the Earth's surface is electrically conductive, and when humans come into direct contact with it, the body absorbs negative electrons. This process helps balance the body's electrical charge, which can significantly reduce inflammation.

The human body functions much like an electrical circuit, requiring a proper balance of ions—charged particles—to maintain optimal physiological processes. When we ground ourselves, negatively charged electrons from the Earth enter our bodies, counteracting the positive charges associated with inflammation. While inflammation is a natural immune response beneficial in acute situations, it becomes harmful when it turns chronic. Chronic inflammation can lead to various health issues, including cardiovascular diseases, diabetes, and neurodegenerative disorders.

Grounding has been shown to reduce chronic inflammation by providing a continuous supply of free electrons, which neutralize free radicals that contribute to oxidative stress. As inflammation decreases, the body's cells can function more effectively, repair themselves, and maintain homeostasis. Grounding supports cellular health in several critical ways. It reduces oxidative stress by absorbing free electrons from the Earth, which neutralize the free radicals that damage cells. This reduction in oxidative stress protects cell membranes, mitochondria, and DNA, allowing cells to operate more efficiently.

Additionally, grounding improves mitochondrial function. Mitochondria, the energy-producing organelles within cells, are particularly vulnerable to damage from oxidative stress. Grounding helps protect mitochondria from free radical damage, supporting ATP (adenosine triphosphate) production and improving overall cellular energy levels. Mitochondria require a stable electrical charge and sufficient electrons to perform their functions efficiently. Grounding also helps balance the autonomic nervous system, reducing sympathetic nervous system activity (responsible for the "fight or flight" response) while enhancing parasympathetic nervous system activity (responsible for relaxation and healing). This balance promotes cellular repair, reduces stress-related inflammation, and supports overall health.

Furthermore, grounding enhances immune function by reducing chronic inflammation and oxidative stress, thereby improving the immune system's ability to fight infections and repair damaged tissues. According to research in *Integrative Medicine: A Clinician's Journal*, grounding increases the production of immune-regulating molecules, supporting the body's ability to heal itself and resist disease. By reconnecting the body with the Earth's natural energy, grounding restores balance at the cellular level and promotes overall health.

The Science of Grounding: Studies Showing How Direct Contact with the Earth Improves Sleep and Decreases Pain

In recent decades, numerous studies have explored the health benefits of grounding. These studies demonstrate that grounding has a significant impact on sleep quality, pain reduction, inflammation, and overall well-being. One well-documented benefit is its ability to reduce inflammation. A study published in *The Journal of Inflammation Research* found that grounding significantly decreased levels of inflammatory markers in the blood, including C-reactive protein (CRP), a key indicator of systemic inflammation. Participants experienced a noticeable reduction in pain and inflammation after grounding sessions, highlighting the immediate effects of this practice on inflammatory responses.

Grounding also improves sleep quality. A study published in *Sleep and Biological Rhythms* examined the effects of grounding on sleep patterns and found that individuals who practiced grounding experienced better sleep quality and fewer disturbances. Participants who used grounding mats reported improved sleep, partly by helping regulate cortisol levels—the hormone responsible for stress. Elevated cortisol levels at night can disrupt sleep, and grounding helped restore normal cortisol rhythms, promoting restful sleep and reducing nighttime awakenings.

Additionally, grounding has been shown to reduce chronic pain, particularly in individuals with musculoskeletal issues. A study published in *The Journal of Alternative and Complementary Medicine* explored the effects of grounding on pain and found that participants who practiced grounding experienced significant pain reduction. By reducing inflammation and improving circulation, grounding allows more oxygen and nutrients to reach affected tissues, supporting cellular repair.

Chronic stress is a major contributor to inflammation and cellular damage. Grounding has been shown to reduce stress levels by shifting the body into a parasympathetic state, promoting relaxation and healing. Research published in *The Journal of Environmental and Public Health* demonstrated that participants who practiced grounding experienced lower cortisol levels and reduced stress, resulting in enhanced emotional well-being.

Practical Tips for Grounding: Simple Methods to Integrate Grounding into Daily Life

Grounding is a simple, natural practice that can easily be incorporated into daily life. It doesn't require special equipment or expensive treatments—just direct contact with the Earth's surface. One of the most effective ways to ground is by walking barefoot on natural surfaces like grass, soil, or sand. Walking barefoot allows your body to absorb electrons from the Earth's surface, helping to balance your body's electrical charge and reduce inflammation.

For those living in urban environments, grounding mats and sheets can simulate direct contact with the Earth. These products connect to a grounding rod or an electrical outlet's grounding port, enabling individuals to remain grounded indoors. This is particularly beneficial for those who spend most of their time indoors or have limited access to natural environments.

Spending time in nature is one of the most effective ways to reconnect with the Earth's energy. Whether hiking, gardening, or simply sitting in a park, being in natural environments allows the body to absorb the Earth's electrons, restoring balance to the cells. Gardening with bare hands also creates a direct connection between the skin and the Earth.

Swimming in natural bodies of water, such as oceans, lakes, or rivers, is another excellent way to ground. Water is a conductor of energy, and immersion in natural water enhances the absorption of the Earth's electrons.

Grounding as a Pathway to Cellular Balance and Health

Grounding is a powerful practice that reconnects us with the Earth's energy, restoring balance at the cellular level and supporting long-term health. By incorporating grounding into our daily routines, we can reduce inflammation, improve sleep, relieve pain, and enhance overall well-being. Scientific research continues to validate the many benefits of grounding, providing compelling evidence that this simple practice can profoundly impact cellular function and promote healing.

As we reconnect with the Earth, we rediscover the ancient wisdom that health, balance, and vitality are all around us, waiting for us to listen to its rhythm.

Conclusion

In summary, grounding serves as a vital connection between our bodies and the Earth, facilitating a natural flow of energy that supports cellular balance and health. By reducing inflammation, enhancing mitochondrial function, and improving overall well-being, grounding offers an accessible way to restore our health in a modern world that is often disconnected from nature. As we move forward, we will explore nutrition for mitochondrial health and how what we eat can further enhance our cellular vitality and energy production.

CHAPTER TEN

Nutrition for Mitochondrial Health

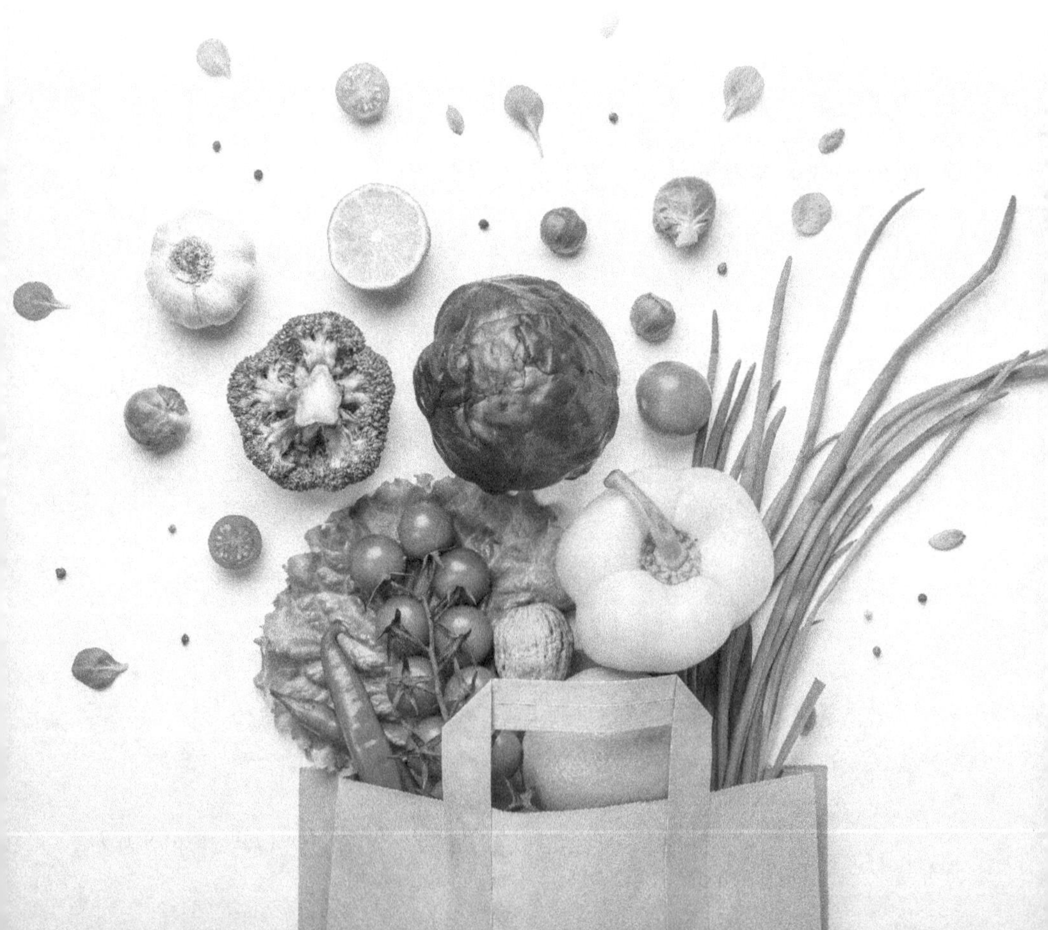

"Let food be thy medicine." —Hippocrates

Hippocrates' famous dictum, "Let food be thy medicine," speaks to the time-less truth that the foods we consume profoundly impact our health and well-being. Today, we understand that food plays a critical role in supporting the function of the mitochondria—the powerhouses of our cells that generate the energy needed for virtually every bodily process. Mitochondria convert the food we eat into adenosine triphosphate (ATP), the molecule that powers cellular activity, growth, and repair. In this chapter, we'll explore how nutrition affects mitochondrial health, identify key nutrients that support mitochondrial function, and discuss the benefits of an anti-inflammatory diet for reducing oxidative stress and promoting cellular healing.

The Role of Diet in Supporting Mitochondrial Function and Cellular Energy

A grass-fed, pasture-raised, clean carnivore diet can be an effective option for supporting mitochondrial health, and it happens to be my personal preference. This diet provides high-quality proteins, healthy fats, and essential nutrients while minimizing exposure to toxins and inflammatory compounds, thereby optimizing cellular energy production and mitochondrial function. Mitochondria are the engines of our cells, responsible for producing the energy necessary for everything from muscle contraction and brain activity to detoxification and immune response. However, these tiny organelles are highly sensitive to environmental stressors, including poor diet, toxins, and oxidative damage. When mitochondria are compromised, energy production declines, leading to fatigue, slower healing, and an increased risk of chronic diseases such as diabetes, neurodegenerative conditions, and cardio-vascular disease.

According to a study published in *Nature Reviews Molecular Cell Biology*, maintaining mitochondrial health is essential for preventing age-related decline and promoting longevity. Diet plays a key role in this process by providing the nutrients mitochondria need to function optimally and protecting them from damage caused by free radicals. Mitochondria generate ATP through oxidative phosphorylation, a process that relies on a steady supply of oxygen, glucose, fatty acids, and specific vitamins and minerals. Without adequate nutrition, mitochondria cannot efficiently produce energy, leading to cellular dysfunction.

In addition to fueling energy production, the right diet can also protect mitochondria from oxidative stress—a condition that occurs when there is an imbalance between free radicals and the body's ability to neutralize them with antioxidants. Oxidative stress is a major contributor to mitochondrial dysfunction, as free radicals can damage mitochondrial DNA and impair ATP production. Over time, this damage can accumulate, leading to inflammation, chronic disease, and accelerated aging. To support mitochondrial health, it's essential to consume a diet rich in nutrient-dense foods that provide the raw materials needed for energy production, as well as antioxidants that protect against oxidative damage. By nourishing the mitochondria, we can boost cellular energy, enhance overall health, and promote long-term vitality.

Grass-Fed, Pasture-Raised, Clean Carnivore Diet and Mitochondrial Health

The grass-fed, pasture-raised, clean carnivore diet is gaining recognition for its potential to support mitochondrial function and cellular energy production. This diet emphasizes consuming animal products that are free from hormones, antibiotics, and toxins, while ensuring the animals were raised on natural diets, leading to more nutrient-dense food. Here's how this diet benefits mitochondrial health:

Grass-fed and pasture-raised meats are rich in high-quality proteins that provide essential amino acids necessary for cellular repair and growth. These proteins support the synthesis of mitochondrial enzymes and proteins, which are vital for energy production. The diet is also abundant in omega-3 fatty acids, conjugated linoleic acid (CLA), and other healthy fats that help maintain the integrity of cell membranes, including the mitochondrial membrane. These fats support mitochondrial function by providing an efficient fuel source, reducing inflammation, and promoting optimal energy production.

Grass-fed meats, particularly organ meats like liver and heart, are rich in Coenzyme Q10 (CoQ10), a compound crucial for mitochondrial energy production. CoQ10 plays a key role in the electron transport chain, which is essential for generating ATP, the primary energy currency of the cell. By consuming these nutrient-dense foods, individuals can enhance mitochondrial function, contributing to improved overall health.

Another significant aspect of the carnivore diet is its ability to reduce inflammatory load. By consuming clean, pasture-raised animal products, this diet minimizes the intake of inflammatory compounds such as antibiotics, hormones, and omega-6 fatty acids typically found in conventionally raised meat. This reduction in inflammation supports healthier mitochondria, as chronic inflammation can hinder mitochondrial function and energy production.

Moreover, grass-fed and pasture-raised meats are more nutrient-dense than conventionally raised meats. They are rich in essential vitamins and minerals, such as B vitamins (B12, B6, and riboflavin), zinc, iron, and selenium—crucial for mitochondrial function and energy metabolism. These nutrients aid in various processes, including the Krebs cycle, which generates ATP within the mitochondria.

The clean carnivore diet also provides ample amounts of carnitine and creatine, both of which are essential for mitochondrial energy metabolism. Carnitine facilitates the transport of fatty acids into the mitochondria for oxidation and energy production, while creatine supports ATP synthesis, particularly during high-energy demands. Additionally, focusing on clean, pasture-raised animal products avoids toxins, preservatives, and additives commonly found in processed meats, thus reducing oxidative stress on mitochondria and allowing them to function more efficiently.

Key Nutrients for Mitochondrial Health

Maintaining optimal mitochondrial function requires a steady supply of specific nutrients that fuel ATP production, protect against oxidative damage, and support cellular repair. Key nutrients for mitochondrial health include antioxidants, B vitamins, carnitine, creatine, CoQ10, and magnesium.

Antioxidants are essential for neutralizing free radicals, protecting mitochondria from oxidative damage. Since mitochondria are the primary source of free radicals, they are particularly vulnerable to oxidative stress. A diet rich in antioxidants helps mitigate this damage and supports mitochondrial function. Vitamin C, a potent antioxidant, protects mitochondria by neutralizing free radicals and plays a crucial role in regenerating other antioxidants, such as vitamin E. Research published in *The American Journal of Clinical Nutrition* indicates that vitamin C supplementation can enhance mitochondrial function, particularly in individuals with oxidative stress-related conditions. Vitamin E also helps safeguard the lipid membranes of cells and mitochondria from oxidative damage. Foods rich in vitamin E include almonds, sunflower seeds, spinach, and avocados.

Glutathione, known as the "master antioxidant," is produced by the body and plays a key role in detoxification and protecting mitochondria from oxidative damage. Higher levels of glutathione are linked to improved mitochondrial efficiency and reduced oxidative stress, as highlighted in Free Radical Biology and Medicine.

CoQ10 is a naturally occurring antioxidant essential for mitochondrial energy production. It is a key component of the electron transport chain, where it helps transfer electrons to generate ATP. CoQ10 also acts as an antioxidant, protecting mitochondria from oxidative damage and promoting cellular repair. According to a study published in *Mitochondrion*, CoQ10 levels decline with age, contributing to reduced mitochondrial function and energy production in aging individuals. Supplementing with CoQ10 has been shown to improve mitochondrial efficiency, reduce fatigue, and boost overall energy levels. Foods rich in CoQ10 include fatty fish (such as salmon and mackerel), organ meats, and whole grains.

Polyphenols, found in foods like berries, green tea, dark chocolate, and red wine, are plant-based antioxidants that protect mitochondria from oxidative damage and improve cellular energy production. Polyphenols also support mitochondrial biogenesis, the process of creating new mitochondria, which is essential for maintaining energy levels and promoting longevity.

B vitamins play a critical role in energy production by acting as cofactors in the mitochondrial pathways that convert carbohydrates, fats, and proteins into ATP. Without sufficient B vitamins, mitochondrial function is compromised, leading to fatigue, cognitive decline, and increased oxidative stress. For example, vitamin B1 (thiamine) is vital for ATP production, while vitamin B12 supports red blood cell formation and nerve health. Foods rich in B vitamins include whole grains, legumes, eggs, dairy products, poultry, and fish.

Carnitine, an amino acid derivative, is essential for transporting fatty acids into the mitochondria, where they are oxidized for energy production. Deficiencies in carnitine can lead to reduced mitochondrial function and increased fatigue, making it especially important for individuals on plant-based diets, who may not get enough from food sources.

Creatine is another crucial nutrient that supports ATP synthesis, particularly during high-energy demands. It helps replenish ATP stores, providing a quick source of energy for muscular contractions and other cellular process-es. Foods rich in creatine include red meat and fish.

Magnesium is an essential mineral involved in numerous biochemical re-actions, particularly those related to energy metabolism. It is crucial for ATP synthesis, helping convert ADP to ATP. Magnesium also stabilizes mitochondrial membranes, which is critical for effective energy production. Research shows that low magnesium levels can decrease mitochondrial ef-ficiency and increase oxidative stress, further impairing energy production. This mineral also has antioxidant properties, helping protect mitochondria from oxidative damage. Foods rich in magnesium include leafy green veg-etables (such as spinach and kale), nuts, seeds, whole grains, and legumes.

The Importance of a Nutrient-Dense, Anti-Inflammatory Diet

Chronic inflammation significantly contributes to mitochondrial dysfunc-tion and cellular damage. An anti-inflammatory diet focuses on foods that reduce inflammation, support mitochondrial health, and promote cellular healing. Key components of this diet include omega-3 fatty acids found in fatty fish (such as salmon and mackerel), flaxseeds, chia seeds, and walnuts. Omega-3s have powerful anti-inflammatory effects and support mitochon-drial function by improving cell membrane fluidity. Leafy green vegetables like spinach, kale, and Swiss chard are packed with antioxidants and vita-mins that reduce inflammation and promote cellular repair, and they also contain magnesium, which is essential for mitochondrial function.

Low-glycemic berries, such as blueberries, strawberries, and raspberries, are rich in polyphenols, particularly anthocyanins, which provide anti-inflammatory and antioxidant effects. Turmeric, which contains curcumin, is known for its anti-inflammatory properties and protects mitochondria from oxidative stress while improving mitochondrial function. Nuts and seeds, including almonds, walnuts, flaxseeds, and chia seeds, offer healthy fats, fiber, and antioxidants that support mitochondrial health.

Recipes for a Mitochondrial Function-Rich, Anti-Inflammatory Diet

To support mitochondrial health, it's essential to include recipes that emphasize nutrient-dense, anti-inflammatory ingredients. Below are a few recipe ideas:

Salmon with Spinach and Quinoa Salad

Ingredients: Salmon fillet, fresh spinach, quinoa, cherry tomatoes, olive oil, lemon, and walnuts.

Preparation: Grill or bake the salmon fillet. Cook quinoa according to package instructions. Toss spinach, quinoa, tomatoes, and walnuts in a bowl. Drizzle with olive oil and lemon juice, and top with the cooked salmon.

Bone Broth Vegetable Soup

Ingredients: Bone broth, carrots, celery, onions, garlic, spinach, and herbs.

Preparation: Sauté onions and garlic until fragrant. Add chopped carrots and celery, followed by the bone broth. Simmer and add spinach just before serving.

Chia Seed Pudding

Ingredients: Chia seeds, almond milk, honey, and fresh berries.
Preparation: Mix chia seeds with almond milk and honey. Let it sit overnight in the fridge. Serve topped with fresh berries.

Turmeric Chicken Stir-Fry

Ingredients: Chicken breast, broccoli, bell peppers, turmeric, garlic, and ginger.
Preparation: Sauté garlic and ginger, then add diced chicken and cook until browned. Add vegetables and turmeric, cooking until the vegetables are tender.

Green Smoothie

Ingredients: Spinach, kale, banana, almond milk, and a scoop of protein powder.
Preparation: Blend all ingredients until smooth for a nutrient-dense breakfast.

7-Day Diet Plan Incorporating Key Nutrients

Day 1:

Breakfast: Scrambled eggs with spinach and avocado.

Lunch: Quinoa salad with cherry tomatoes, cucumbers, and feta cheese.

Dinner: Grilled salmon with steamed broccoli and sweet potato.

Day 2:

Breakfast: Chia seed pudding topped with fresh berries.

Lunch: Bone broth soup with mixed vegetables.

Dinner: Grass-fed beef stir-fry with bell peppers and brown rice.

Day 3:

Breakfast: Smoothie with kale, banana, and almond milk.

Lunch: Turkey lettuce wraps with avocado and salsa.

Dinner: Baked chicken thighs with roasted Brussels sprouts and quinoa.

Day 4:

Breakfast: Greek yogurt with honey, walnuts, and blueberries.

Lunch: Spinach and feta-stuffed chicken breast with asparagus.

Dinner: Lentil soup with carrots and celery.

Day 5:

Breakfast: Omelet with mushrooms and tomatoes.

Lunch: Mixed greens salad with grilled shrimp and vinaigrette.

Dinner: Zucchini noodles with turkey meatballs and marinara sauce.

Day 6:

Breakfast: Smoothie with spinach, protein powder, and almond butter.

Lunch: Quinoa and black bean bowl with salsa and avocado.

Dinner: Roast pork tenderloin with cauliflower mash and green beans.

Day 7:

Breakfast: Pancakes made with almond flour and topped with berries.

Lunch: Chicken Caesar salad with homemade dressing.

Dinner: Grilled lamb chops with roasted root vegetables.

By focusing on a nutrient-dense, anti-inflammatory diet that includes a variety of high-quality foods, individuals can support mitochondrial health, optimize cellular function, and reduce the risk of chronic diseases. Incorporating these nutrient-rich foods into your daily meals ensures the body receives the essential building blocks for promoting mitochondrial function and overall health. This commitment to nutrition reflects the wisdom of Hippocrates, who understood the profound impact food has on our well-being.

7-Day Strict Carnivore Diet Plan

Day 1:

Breakfast: Scrambled eggs cooked in grass-fed butter, topped with crispy bacon.

Lunch: Grilled ribeye steak seasoned with salt and pepper.

Dinner: Baked salmon fillet with a side of bone broth.

Day 2:

Breakfast: Omelet made with three eggs, shredded cheese, and diced ham.

Lunch: Ground beef patties with bone marrow.

Dinner: Roasted chicken thighs with skin, served with chicken liver pâté.

Day 3:

Breakfast: Beef liver sautéed in butter, served with sunny-side-up eggs.

Lunch: Grilled pork chops seasoned with herbs and spices.

Dinner: Rack of lamb roasted with garlic and rosemary.

Day 4:

Breakfast: Breakfast sausages made from grass-fed pork.

Lunch: Shrimp sautéed in butter, seasoned with lemon zest.

Dinner: Whole roasted duck, served with duck fat drizzled over it.

Day 5:

Breakfast: Hard-boiled eggs, served with homemade beef jerky.

Lunch: Brisket slow-cooked until tender.

Dinner: Seared tuna steak, garnished with a sprinkle of sea salt.

Day 6:

Breakfast: Soft-boiled eggs, served with slices of smoked salmon.

Lunch: Beef tongue, cooked until tender and sliced thin.

Dinner: Grilled bison burgers topped with cheese.

Day 7:

Breakfast: Poached eggs over slices of pork belly.

Lunch: Venison steaks cooked medium-rare.

Dinner: Sautéed scallops in butter, with a side of crab legs.

Nutritional Considerations

- **High Protein Intake**: Aim for 30-50 grams of protein per meal to support muscle maintenance and energy levels, especially when paired with intermittent fasting.
- **Healthy Fats**: Include sources of healthy fats from animal products, such as bone marrow and duck fat, to maintain cell membrane integrity and support mitochondrial function.
- **Essential Nutrients**: This carnivore diet provides vital nutrients like CoQ10 from organ meats, B vitamins from eggs and meat, and carnitine from red meat, all of which are crucial for mitochondrial energy production.
- **Anti-Inflammatory Properties**: Grass-fed and pasture-raised animal products are typically lower in inflammatory omega-6 fatty acids, helping reduce systemic inflammation and support cellular health.

This 7-day strict carnivore diet plan emphasizes the consumption of nutrient-dense animal products, ensuring a focus on mitochondrial health. By following this plan, individuals can optimize energy levels, reduce inflammation, and support overall well-being through a tailored, nutrient-rich approach that aligns with health goals.

Conclusion

By focusing on a nutrient-dense, anti-inflammatory diet that incorporates high-quality foods, individuals can significantly support mitochondrial health, optimize cellular function, and reduce the risk of chronic diseases. This chapter highlights the crucial role nutrition plays in cellular health, emphasizing that what we put into our bodies directly impacts how our cells function.

As Hippocrates wisely stated, "Let food be thy medicine." This ancient wisdom remains ever relevant today. The choices we make at every meal can either nourish or hinder our health. Consuming processed foods high in sugars, unhealthy fats, and additives—essentially "junk"—leads to poor health outcomes like fatigue, inflammation, and an increased risk of chronic diseases, all stemming from our nutritional choices.

Conversely, by prioritizing whole, nutrient-dense foods, we empower our bodies to thrive. It is essential to make smart dietary choices that align with our health goals while minimizing unhealthy options that can lead to cellular dysfunction. Understanding the profound relationship between diet and mitochondrial function enables us to take actionable steps toward better health.

In conclusion, we must remain vigilant and intentional about our food choices, recognizing that they are foundational to our cellular health. Our mitochondria, which power every cell in our bodies, are significantly influenced by our diet. Let us commit to a lifestyle that embraces nutritious foods, supporting our bodies in their quest for energy, vitality, and longevity. By choosing wisely, we not only enhance our mitochondrial health but also cultivate a better quality of life overall. As we transition into the next chapter on exercise and cellular regeneration, remember that nutrition and physical activity go hand in hand. Just as the food we consume fuels our bodies, regular exercise is vital for maintaining mitochondrial function and promoting overall cellular health. Together, these two components form the cornerstone of a vibrant, healthy life.

CHAPTER ELEVEN

Exercise and Cellular Regeneration

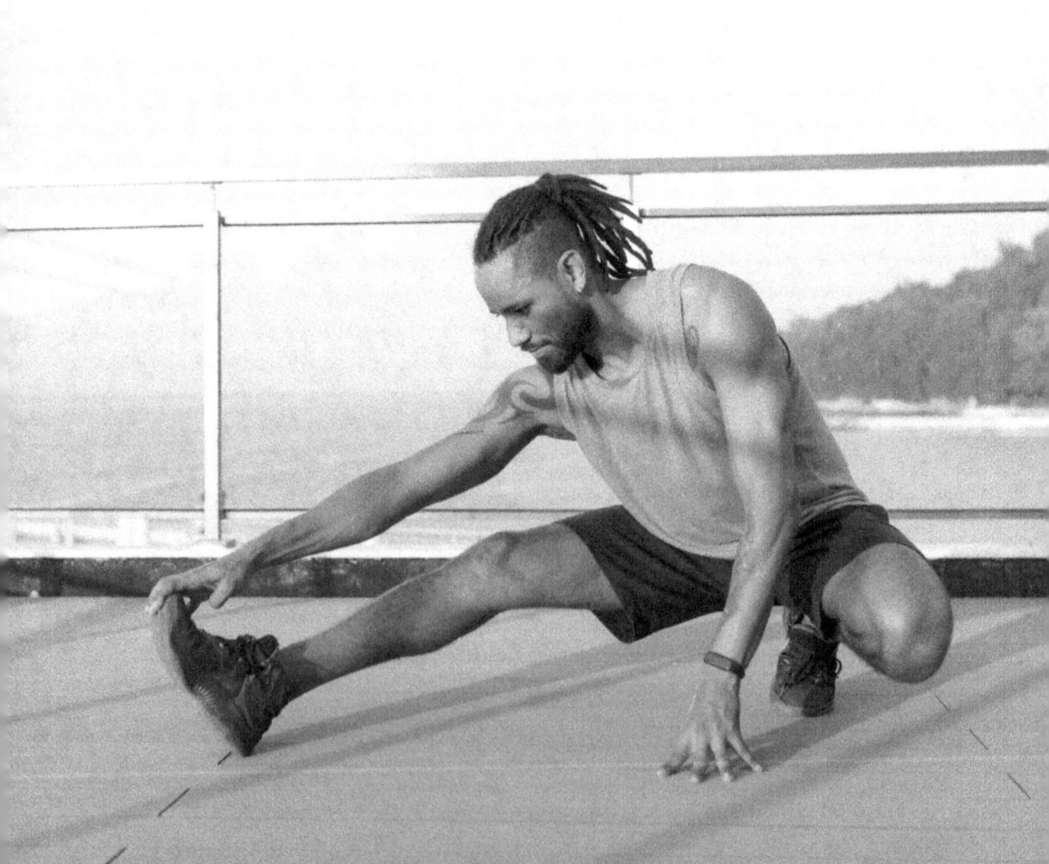

"Movement is medicine." This simple yet profound quote highlights the powerful impact that physical activity has on our health and well-being. Just as food nourishes our bodies, movement stimulates cellular processes that promote healing, repair, and regeneration. Exercise is not just a tool for maintaining physical fitness; it is a key component of cellular health, helping to optimize mitochondrial function, reduce inflammation, and enhance overall longevity. In this chapter, we will explore how exercise stimulates cellular regeneration, discuss the specific benefits of high-intensity interval training (HIIT) for mitochondrial health, and emphasize the importance of balancing movement with rest to ensure optimal recovery and cellular healing.

How Physical Activity Stimulates Cellular Repair and Regeneration

The human body is designed for movement, and physical activity is essential for maintaining health at the cellular level. Exercise activates a range of biological processes that promote the repair and regeneration of cells, tissues, and organs. Think of your body as a busy factory, where physical activity acts as a maintenance crew, fixing machines and ensuring everything runs smoothly. Just as regular maintenance prevents breakdowns and enhances efficiency, consistent exercise supports cellular function and overall health.

At the core of the relationship between movement and cellular regeneration is the concept of hormesis—the process by which low levels of stress stimulate cellular adaptation and repair. When we engage in physical activity, particularly high-intensity or resistance-based exercises, we create mild stress on the body. This stress triggers the release of signaling molecules that promote the repair of damaged cells, stimulate the growth of new cells, and enhance the body's ability to adapt to future challenges. It's like a workout for your cells: just as lifting weights strengthens muscles, the stress of exercise strengthens cellular resilience.

One of the most important systems affected by exercise is the mitochondria—the energy-producing organelles within our cells. Think of mitochondria as power plants that generate the energy (in the form of ATP) fueling cellular processes. Just as power plants need regular upgrades and maintenance to operate efficiently, our mitochondria require regular exercise to function at their best. Exercise enhances mitochondrial function by increasing the number of mitochondria in each cell (a process called mitochondrial biogenesis) and improving the efficiency of existing mitochondria. Research published in *Cell Metabolism* has shown that regular physical activity enhances mitochondrial health by boosting ATP production, reducing oxidative stress, and improving the cell's ability to detoxify itself.

In addition to boosting mitochondrial function, exercise stimulates the release of growth factors like brain-derived neurotrophic factor (BDNF) and insulin-like growth factor 1 (IGF-1), both of which support cellular repair and regeneration. Think of BDNF as a gardener nurturing the growth of neurons, while IGF-1 acts like fertilizer promoting muscle repair. These growth factors not only aid cellular recovery following exercise but also protect against age-related decline in cell function.

Exercise also plays a critical role in reducing inflammation, a major contributor to cellular damage and dysfunction. A study published in *The Journal of Physiology* found that regular physical activity reduces the levels of pro-inflammatory cytokines and increases the production of anti-inflammatory molecules. This reduction in inflammation supports the body's natural healing processes, enabling cells to repair themselves more effectively and reducing the risk of chronic disease. Ultimately, movement stimulates many cellular processes that promote repair, regeneration, and adaptation.

How High-Intensity Interval Training (HIIT) Boosts Mitochondrial Health

High-intensity interval training (HIIT) has gained widespread popularity for its ability to deliver maximum benefits in a short amount of time. HIIT involves alternating between short bursts of intense activity and brief periods of rest or lower-intensity movement. This form of exercise challenges the body in unique ways, triggering powerful adaptations that enhance mitochondrial function, improve cardiovascular health, and promote fat loss. The benefits of HIIT for mitochondrial health are particularly significant, as this type of training can significantly boost both the efficiency and capacity of the mitochondria.

Mitochondrial Biogenesis

One of the most notable benefits of HIIT is its ability to stimulate mitochondrial biogenesis—the process by which new mitochondria are produced within cells. A study published in *The American Journal of Physiology* shows that HIIT increases the expression of peroxisome proliferator-activated receptor gamma coactivator 1-alpha (PGC-1α), a key regulator of mitochondrial biogenesis. Imagine your cells as a factory that needs more assembly lines to meet growing production demands. HIIT essentially adds new assembly lines, increasing energy production and overall metabolic efficiency. As more mitochondria are produced, the cell's capacity to generate energy increases, enhancing overall metabolic function and reducing the risk of fatigue and cellular dysfunction. Mitochondrial biogenesis is especially important as we age, as mitochondrial function naturally declines with time. By engaging in HIIT, individuals can stimulate the production of new mitochondria, helping to counteract the effects of aging and maintain cellular vitality.

Improved Mitochondrial Efficiency

In addition to increasing the number of mitochondria, HIIT also improves the efficiency of existing mitochondria. This means that the mitochondria can produce more ATP with less oxygen, enabling cells to function more efficiently, even under stress. A study published in *The Journal of Applied Physiology* found that HIIT enhances the activity of enzymes involved in the electron transport chain—the process by which mitochondria produce ATP. This can be likened to a more efficient assembly line in a factory, one that not only produces more products but also does so with fewer raw materials. As a result, individuals who engage in HIIT experience improved energy levels, reduced oxidative stress, and enhanced endurance.

Reduction in Oxidative Stress

Oxidative stress occurs when there's an imbalance between the production of free radicals and the body's ability to neutralize them with antioxidants. Free radicals can damage mitochondria, impairing their ability to produce energy and leading to cellular dysfunction. HIIT has been shown to reduce oxidative stress by enhancing the body's natural antioxidant defenses.

Research published in *Free Radical Biology and Medicine* suggests that HIIT increases the activity of antioxidant enzymes such as superoxide dismutase (SOD) and glutathione peroxidase, which protect mitochondria from oxidative damage. Think of HIIT as a shield that not only protects mitochondria from incoming attacks but also strengthens the body's defense mechanisms against oxidative stress. By reducing oxidative stress, HIIT improves mitochondrial function and supports overall cellular health, reducing the risk of chronic diseases associated with oxidative damage, such as heart disease and neurodegenerative conditions.

Enhanced Fat Metabolism

One of the unique benefits of HIIT is its ability to enhance fat metabolism, allowing the body to burn fat more efficiently for energy. During high-intensity intervals, the body primarily relies on glycogen (stored carbohydrates) for fuel. However, during the recovery periods, the body shifts to burning fat as its primary energy source. This process, known as excess post-exercise oxygen consumption (EPOC), continues for hours after the workout, resulting in increased fat burning and improved metabolic flexibility. Research published in *The Journal of Obesity* shows that individuals who engage in

HIIT experience greater reductions in body fat and improved insulin sensitivity compared to those who engage in steady-state cardio. This enhanced fat metabolism not only supports weight management but also improves mitochondrial function, as mitochondria are responsible for breaking down fats and converting them into ATP.

Cardiovascular Benefits

In addition to its positive effects on mitochondrial health, HIIT offers significant benefits for cardiovascular health. HIIT improves heart function, increases lung capacity, and enhances blood flow—factors that all contribute to better oxygen delivery to the cells. As more oxygen is delivered to the mitochondria, ATP production increases, enabling cells to generate energy more efficiently. A study published in *The Journal of Sports Medicine and Physical Fitness* indicates that HIIT increases VO2 max, a measure of the body's ability to use oxygen during exercise. Think of VO2 max as the body's engine capacity: higher levels mean your engine runs more efficiently and can sustain higher levels of activity for longer periods. Higher VO2 max levels are associated with improved endurance, better cardiovascular health, and enhanced mitochondrial function.

Balancing Rest and Movement: Importance of Recovery for Cellular Healing

While exercise is essential for promoting cellular repair and regeneration, it is equally important to balance physical activity with adequate rest and recovery. Overtraining or failing to allow sufficient time for recovery can lead to cellular damage, increased inflammation, and impaired healing. Recovery is the period during which the body repairs the microtears in muscle fibers, restores energy stores, and regenerates cells. Without proper recovery, the body becomes more susceptible to injury, fatigue, and cellular dysfunction.

Sleep is one of the most critical factors in the recovery process. During sleep, the body undergoes numerous repair and regeneration processes that are essential for maintaining cellular health. A study published in *Sleep Medicine Reviews* shows that deep sleep, also known as slow-wave sleep, is the stage during which the body releases growth hormone—a key driver of tissue repair and muscle recovery. Sleep also supports mitochondrial function by reducing oxidative stress and promoting the removal of damaged cells through a process called autophagy.

Think of sleep as the nightly maintenance crew for your factory, ensuring everything is in working order for the next day. Inadequate sleep can impair these repair processes, leading to reduced athletic performance, slower recovery times, and an increased risk of injury. Ensuring adequate, high-quality sleep is essential for supporting cellular regeneration and optimizing the benefits of exercise.

Active Recovery

While rest is important, incorporating active recovery—low-intensity movement such as walking, yoga, or stretching—can enhance circulation, reduce muscle soreness, and support cellular healing. Active recovery increases blood flow to the muscles, delivering oxygen and nutrients that aid tissue repair, while also helping to remove waste products like lactic acid. According to a study published in *The Journal of Strength and Conditioning Research*, active recovery has been shown to reduce muscle soreness and improve flexibility, allowing individuals to recover more quickly between high-intensity workouts. Activities such as light jogging, swimming, or gentle yoga can help promote cellular healing while maintaining physical activity.

Hydration and Nutrition for Recovery

Proper hydration and nutrition are crucial for supporting recovery and cellular regeneration. Water is essential for maintaining cellular function, as it helps transport nutrients to cells and remove metabolic waste. Dehydration can impair cellular repair and increase the risk of injury. In addition to staying hydrated, consuming nutrient-dense foods that support recovery is equally important. Protein, in particular, plays a vital role in muscle repair, providing the amino acids needed to rebuild damaged tissues. Research published in *The American Journal of Clinical Nutrition* shows that consuming protein-rich foods after exercise enhances muscle recovery and promotes the regeneration of new cells. Including anti-inflammatory foods such as leafy greens, berries, and fatty fish can further support cellular healing by reducing inflammation and oxidative stress. These foods provide antioxidants and nutrients that protect cells from damage and enhance the body's natural repair processes.

Incorporating Rest Days

While consistent exercise is important for maintaining health, it's equally crucial to incorporate rest days into your fitness routine. Rest days give your body the opportunity to recover from the stress of exercise, repair damaged tissues, and restore energy levels. According to a study in *The Journal of Sports*

Sciences, overtraining can lead to increased levels of cortisol, the body's primary stress hormone, which can impair recovery and increase the risk of injury. Scheduling one or two rest days per week allows your body to fully recover, reducing the risk of burnout and ensuring that your cells have the time they need to regenerate.

Mind-Body Practices for Recovery

Incorporating mind-body practices such as meditation, deep breathing, or gentle stretching can enhance recovery by reducing stress and promoting relaxation. A study published in *Frontiers in Human Neuroscience* indicates that meditation and mindfulness practices have been shown to lower cortisol levels, improve sleep quality, and enhance overall recovery. These practices activate the parasympathetic nervous system, which promotes relaxation and supports cellular repair. By incorporating such practices into your recovery routine, you can further optimize the body's natural healing processes and maximize the benefits of exercise.

Conclusion

Exercise has the power to revitalize our cells, boost energy, and improve our overall health. Whether you prefer high-intensity interval training or more relaxed forms of physical activity, movement sets off a chain reaction of biological processes that help repair cells, reduce inflammation, and promote longevity. However, it's crucial to balance exercise with adequate rest and recovery to maximize these benefits and avoid cellular damage. By combining high-intensity workouts with active recovery, proper hydration, healthy eating, and mindfulness practices, you can support cell regeneration and feel your best. As the saying goes, "Movement is medicine"—when we move with purpose and balance, we give our cells the opportunity to heal, regenerate, and flourish.

As we transition into the next chapter, we will explore the profound effects of meditation, prayer, and mindfulness on our cellular health. These practices not only promote mental clarity and emotional stability but also have significant physiological benefits that can enhance our overall well-being. Just as movement is vital for cellular function, cultivating a mindful approach to life can further support our health, fostering deep relaxation and inner peace that complements our physical efforts. Together, exercise and mindfulness form a holistic approach to health, fostering resilience at both cellular and mental levels.

CHAPTER TWELVE

Meditation, Prayer, and Mindfulness

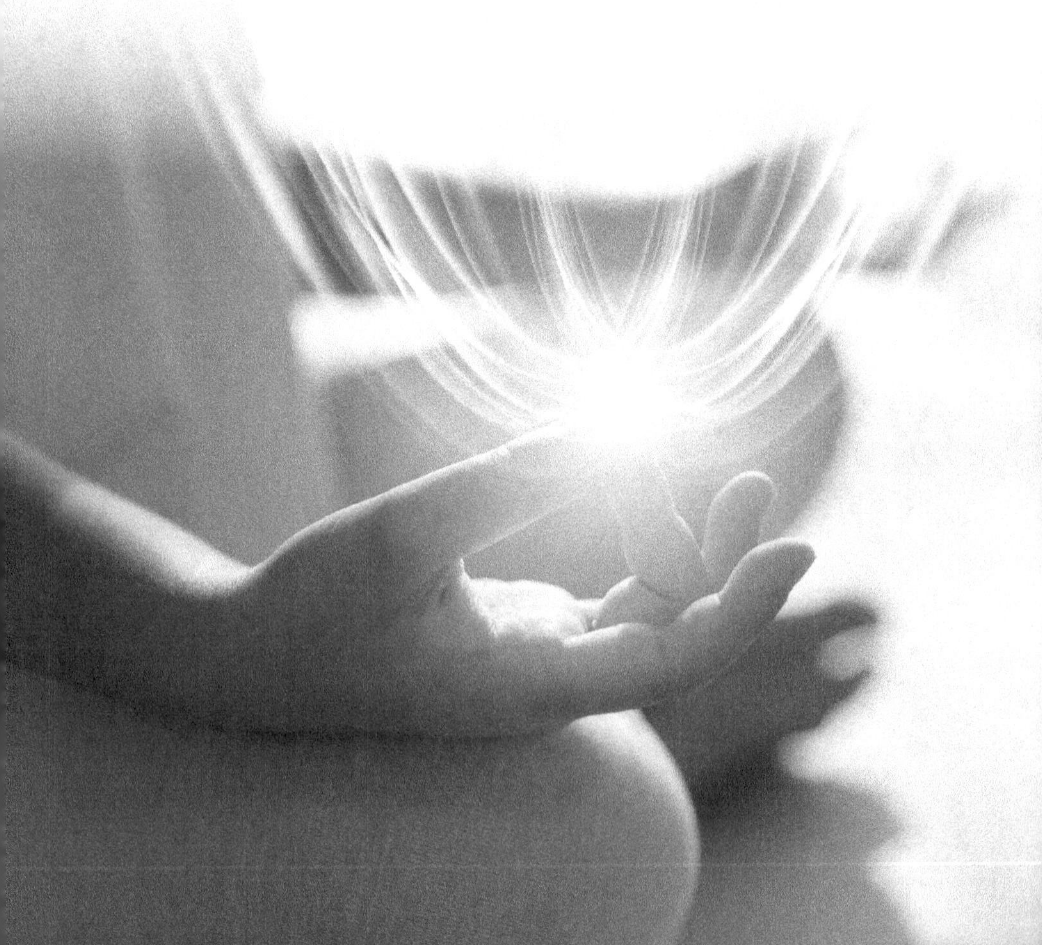

Rumi's timeless wisdom speaks to an essential truth: in the stillness of our inner lives, profound healing can occur. Today, as we navigate constant demands, carving out time for inner peace through prayer, meditation, and mindfulness has become more crucial than ever. These practices go beyond mental clarity; they harmonize our physical, mental, and spiritual selves, nurturing every cell in our body and promoting Cellular Vitality. As scientific evidence grows, it confirms what spiritual traditions have long known: our inner lives profoundly influence our physical health. The mind, body, and soul are not separate; they interact in ways that impact cellular function, repair, and overall well-being.

The Profound Impact of Prayer on Cellular Health

Prayer offers refuge and strength in times of stress, acting as a powerful bridge between the mind and body. For those of faith, prayer is more than a calming ritual; it's a conversation with God—a time to surrender burdens, seek guidance, and cultivate gratitude. Scriptures such as "I can do all things through Christ who strengthens me" (Philippians 4:13) and "For I will restore health to you, and your wounds I will heal, declares the Lord" (Jeremiah 30:17) emphasize the healing and strength available through faith.

From a scientific perspective, prayer's impact on cellular health is linked to the body's parasympathetic nervous system, the "rest and repair" mechanism. When we pray, our bodies reduce the production of cortisol, a stress hormone that can disrupt cellular function, promote inflammation, and cause oxidative stress. This connection between prayer and stress reduction has been well-documented. Research published in *Biological Psychiatry* demonstrates that regular prayer or meditation lowers cortisol levels, which, in turn, supports cellular repair and regeneration.

Imagine each cell in your body as a finely tuned instrument in an orchestra. Stress and cortisol disrupt this harmony, but prayer acts as a conductor, realigning each part and restoring balance. Prayer also stimulates the release of dopamine, a neurochemical that fosters calm, focus, and emotional resilience. This shift not only enhances our sense of peace but also signals to every cell that it's safe to relax and regenerate. Studies suggest that this calming effect enables the immune system to function more efficiently, redirecting resources toward healing rather than defending against stress-related damage.

Meditation's Role in Slowing Cellular Aging

Meditation has been practiced across cultures for thousands of years, but modern research now sheds light on its effects at a cellular level. One of the most remarkable findings is meditation's impact on telomeres—the protective caps at the ends of chromosomes that play a vital role in cellular aging. Studies published in Psychoneuroendocrinology reveal that regular meditation can help maintain telomere length, effectively slowing the cellular aging process.

Telomeres function much like the plastic tips on shoelaces; they prevent DNA from fraying and losing integrity. As telomeres wear down over time, cells become more prone to aging and programmed cell death. However, meditation appears to slow the rate at which telomeres shorten. Imagine telomeres as the biological "clock" of your cells. Each time a cell divides, telomeres shorten slightly, eventually leading to cellular aging. Meditation, however, has been found to protect these telomeres, preserving cellular integrity and extending cellular lifespan. A study cited in *Biological Psychiatry* showed that individuals who meditated regularly had longer telomeres than non-meditators, suggesting that meditation helps protect our cells from the toll of stress and oxidative damage. This resilience allows cells to focus on repair and function optimally, promoting a state of Cellular Vitality that radiates throughout the body.

Meditation's impact extends beyond telomeres. By engaging the brain's relaxation response, meditation shifts the autonomic nervous system into a parasympathetic state, reducing blood pressure, heart rate, and levels of stress hormones. This calming effect enables cells to divert resources from emergency responses to essential repair functions, creating an environment where healing and resilience flourish.

Mindfulness and the Power of Present Awareness

Mindfulness—the practice of staying present and fully engaged in the moment—plays a unique role in supporting cellular health. When practiced regularly, mindfulness helps break cycles of worry and regret, allowing us to approach life's challenges with clarity and calm. Research published in *Applied Psychophysiology and Biofeedback* shows that mindfulness increases heart rate variability (HRV), a marker of adaptability and cardiovascular resilience. Higher HRV is associated with improved stress management, lower inflammation, and better cellular health.

Mindfulness acts as a stabilizing rhythm for the body, much like a river flowing smoothly and nourishing every cell. This rhythmic calm allows cells to repair, regenerate, and function optimally. Practicing gratitude—a core aspect of mindfulness—has been shown to reduce levels of pro-inflammatory cytokines, proteins linked to chronic inflammation and cellular damage. By shifting our focus to gratitude, we create a cellular environment where repair mechanisms are prioritized and stress responses minimized. Studies in Emotion highlight how gratitude reduces inflammation and promotes immune health, allowing cells to function in a state of peace and resilience.

In practical terms, mindfulness can be seen as a natural anti-inflammatory practice. By cultivating awareness of the present moment, we avoid the physiological effects of stress-induced inflammation. Instead, we support our body's healing processes by signaling safety and calm. Mindfulness invites the body into a restorative state, where cells focus on longevity and health rather than responding to perceived threats.

Gratitude's Influence on Cellular Function

Practicing gratitude further enhances the effects of prayer and mindfulness. When we focus on gratitude, we communicate a sense of safety and fulfillment to our cells, creating an environment conducive to healing. Studies published in Personality and Individual Differences show that gratitude significantly lowers cortisol levels and reduces inflammation. The regular practice of gratitude can lead to lasting changes in the body's stress response, promoting resilience and reducing cellular aging.

Picture gratitude as a nutrient for the soul—one that feeds each cell with messages of safety and peace. Gratitude amplifies the effects of mindfulness and prayer, creating a cumulative impact that enhances cellular health. By fostering gratitude, we nourish a mental state that supports physical resilience and reduces the wear and tear of daily stress on our cells.

Prayer and the Divine Design for Healing

For those of faith, prayer is a moment of profound surrender, a release from the burdens of control. By entrusting our worries to a higher power, we shift our mindset, creating space for peace and physiological healing. Research on the effects of prayer has shown that it can improve immune function, lower blood pressure, and reduce inflammation. In prayer, we align with a divine design for healing, promoting a mental state of peace that translates into physical well-being.

Studies show that prayer activates the vagus nerve, stimulating the parasympathetic response that lowers heart rate and promotes relaxation. As the vagus nerve influences inflammatory processes, prayer contributes to a decrease in pro-inflammatory cytokines, which are implicated in chronic diseases and cellular damage. Each time we pray, we engage in an act of self-healing, enabling the body to enter a state of repair. This practice reminds us of the divine blueprint for health, encouraging our cells to respond in alignment with our inherent capacity for healing.

Prayer invites us to connect with a force beyond ourselves, instilling faith that we are supported and guiding our cells into a restorative state. When combined with gratitude, prayer can enhance cellular health by creating a symbiotic relationship between mind and body. Each prayer echoes through our cells, reinforcing their ability to heal and regenerate.

Embracing the Divine Power of the Mind-Body-Soul Connection

The synergy between prayer, meditation, mindfulness, and gratitude creates a powerful foundation for cellular health. These practices align the mind, body, and soul, fostering a healing environment within us that science now affirms. When we engage in these practices regularly, we amplify our body's natural healing abilities, allowing every cell to function in harmony and resilience.

The journey of Cellular Vitality is about embracing the interconnectedness of mind, body, and soul. When we pray, meditate, and practice mindfulness, we send a message to every cell: you are safe, you are loved, you are resilient. This inner harmony extends outward, promoting health, resilience, and vitality. As we tune our inner lives, we foster Cellular Vitality that strengthens our well-being, fortifying us against stress and supporting long-term health.

Moving Forward: Supplements in Cellular Health

In the next chapter, we will explore how specific supplements can enhance cellular health, complementing the resilience cultivated through prayer, meditation, and mindfulness. Together, these practices and nutrients form a holistic approach to health that is both scientifically grounded and spiritually enriching. Embracing these pathways invites a life of Cellular Vitality, where each cell thrives in harmony with the mind, body, and soul.

CHAPTER THIRTEEN

The Role of Supplements in Cellular Health

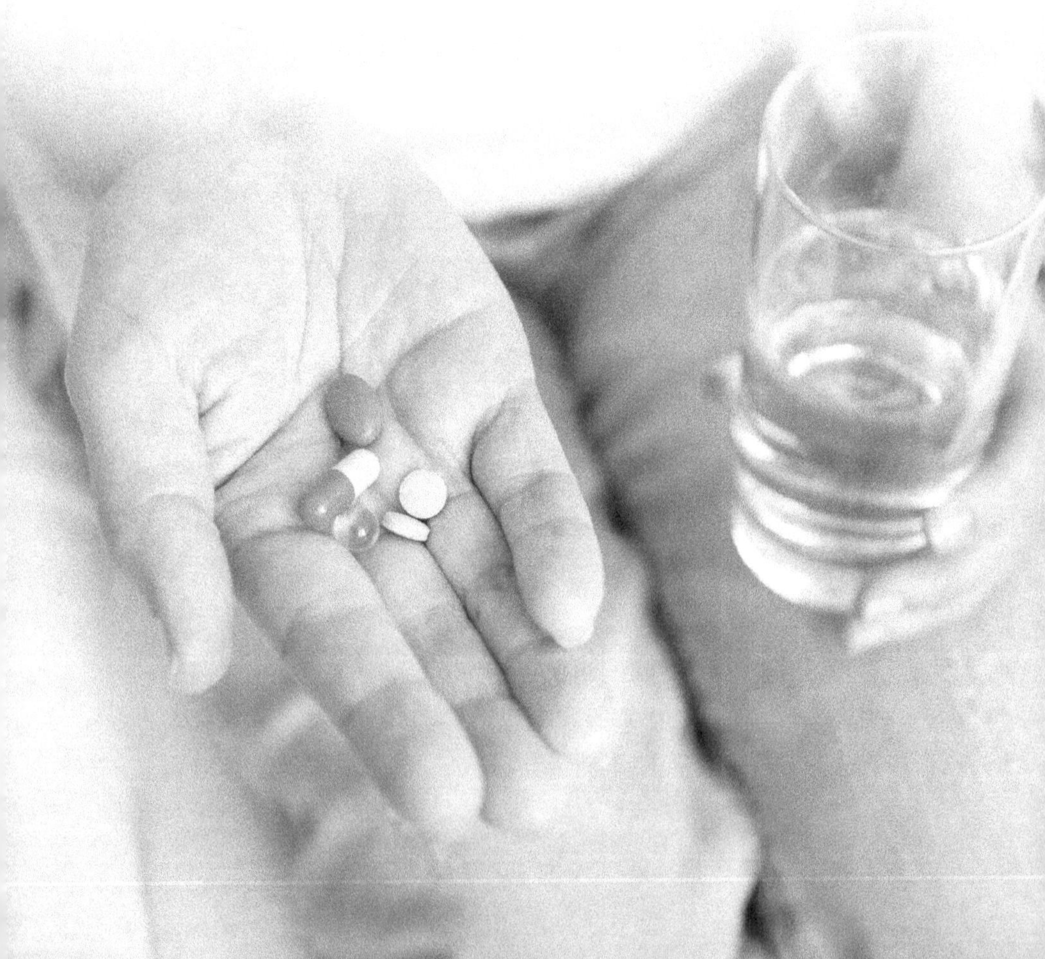

"Nourish your body, and it will serve you well." —Unknown

The human body is a remarkable system capable of healing, repairing, and regenerating itself when given the proper support. This chapter explores how supplements play a critical role in optimizing cellular health—especially when a balanced diet alone is insufficient due to modern lifestyles, environmental stressors, or the natural aging process. These supplements help fill nutritional gaps, combat oxidative stress, and promote energy production, cellular repair, and overall vitality.

Supplements Categorized by Function

To maintain optimal health, cellular functions must be supported by both diet and, in many cases, supplements. Cellular energy production, cell membrane integrity, and the internal environment within which cells operate—often referred to as the "cellular terrain"—are all vital aspects of cellular health. Modern lifestyles, environmental stressors, and aging can compromise these cellular functions.

Research-backed supplements can help fill nutritional gaps, optimize cellular processes, and combat oxidative stress, improving overall health. This section will explore a wide range of supplements categorized by their function: cellular energy production, cell membrane health, and cellular terrain health. Each supplement is supported by scientific studies, ensuring evidence-based recommendations.

1. Cellular Energy Production

Cellular energy production takes place primarily in the mitochondria, where ATP (adenosine triphosphate) is synthesized. As we age, mitochondrial function declines, leading to reduced energy levels, increased fatigue, and higher risks of chronic diseases. The following supplements support mitochondrial health and improve ATP production, enhancing overall energy levels:

Coenzyme Q10 (CoQ10)

CoQ10 is a naturally occurring antioxidant found in the mitochondria of every cell, playing a crucial role in ATP production through the electron transport chain. CoQ10 levels naturally decline with age, particularly affecting high-energy-demand organs like the heart and brain. Studies have shown that CoQ10 supplementation can significantly improve mitochondrial function and reduce oxidative stress.

A study published in *Biofactors* demonstrated that CoQ10 supplementation improved symptoms of chronic fatigue and enhanced mitochondrial bioenergetics in patients with fibromyalgia. Furthermore, research in *The Journal of Clinical Lipidology* revealed that CoQ10 reduced muscle pain associated with statin use, suggesting its protective role in muscle and mitochondrial function.

NAD+ is an essential coenzyme involved in redox reactions that generate ATP. NAD+ levels decline with age, contributing to reduced mitochondrial function and cellular energy. Supplementing with NAD+ precursors, such as nicotinamide riboside (NR) and nicotinamide mononucleotide (NMN), has been shown to restore NAD+ levels, boost energy, and enhance longevity. Research published in *Nature Communications* demonstrated that NR supplementation increased NAD+ levels, improved mitochondrial biogenesis, and enhanced muscle function in aging adults. Another study showed that restoring NAD+ levels through NMN supplementation improved mitochondrial function and reduced age-related physiological decline in animal models.

L-Carnitine

L-Carnitine plays a crucial role in transporting fatty acids into the mitochondria, where they are oxidized for energy production. This is especially important for muscle cells during physical activity, as fatty acids are a key energy source. Studies have shown that L-Carnitine supplementation improves endurance and reduces recovery time after exercise. A clinical trial published in The American Journal of Clinical Nutrition found that L-Carnitine supplementation significantly improved exercise performance and reduced post-exercise muscle soreness by enhancing mitochondrial fatty acid oxidation. In addition, a study about metabolism revealed that L-Carnitine supplementation helped patients with chronic fatigue syndrome improve their overall energy levels.

Alpha-Lipoic Acid (ALA) is both a cofactor for mitochondrial enzymes involved in energy production and a potent antioxidant that protects mitochondria from oxidative damage. ALA has been shown to improve mitochondrial function and reduce oxidative stress, particularly in patients with metabolic disorders. A study published in *Diabetes Care* demonstrated that ALA supplementation improved insulin sensitivity, reduced oxidative stress, and enhanced mitochondrial function in patients with type 2 diabetes. Additionally, a meta-analysis published in Frontiers in Pharmacology confirmed that ALA effectively supports energy metabolism and reduces oxidative stress in metabolic syndrome.

D-Ribose

D-Ribose is a simple sugar that forms the backbone of ATP, making it essential for energy recovery. Supplementation with D-Ribose has been shown to enhance energy production, particularly in individuals suffering from chronic fatigue or during post-exercise recovery. In a clinical study published in *The Journal of Alternative and Complementary Medicine*, patients with fibromyalgia and chronic fatigue syndrome reported significant improvements in energy levels and reduced pain after D-Ribose supplementation. These results suggest that D-Ribose accelerates energy recovery and enhances cellular repair.

Magnesium

Magnesium is essential for more than 300 biochemical reactions, including those involved in ATP production. It acts as a cofactor for enzymes that facilitate energy metabolism, and magnesium deficiency is associated with fatigue and muscle weakness. A study published in *Magnesium Research* found that magnesium supplementation improved mitochondrial function and increased energy production in individuals with chronic fatigue. The study emphasized magnesium's importance in maintaining overall cellular energy.

Creatine Monohydrate

Creatine is known for its role in regenerating ATP in muscle cells during short bursts of high-intensity activity. Supplementation with creatine has been shown to improve strength, power, and endurance by maintaining adequate ATP levels during exercise. A review in *The Journal of the International Society of Sports Nutrition* highlighted that creatine monohydrate significantly enhances athletic performance and muscle mass by increasing the availability of phosphocreatine, which helps regenerate ATP during physical exertion.

Pyrroloquinoline Quinone (PQQ)

PQQ is a potent antioxidant that stimulates mitochondrial biogenesis, increasing the number of mitochondria in cells. This enhances energy production and protects cells from oxidative damage. Research published in *The Journal of Clinical Biochemistry and Nutrition* found that PQQ supplementation improved energy metabolism and reduced markers of oxidative stress in older adults. PQQ's ability to support mitochondrial biogenesis makes it particularly beneficial for health and longevity.

Taurine

Taurine plays a key role in regulating calcium levels within cells, supporting mitochondrial function, and protecting cells from oxidative stress. Studies suggest that taurine supplementation enhances energy levels and supports tissue repair, particularly in the heart and muscles. A study published in *Advances in Experimental Medicine and Biology* found that taurine supplementation improved mitochondrial function and energy production, especially in aging individuals with cardiovascular conditions.

MSM (Methylsulfonylmethane)

Methylsulfonylmethane (MSM) is an organic sulfur compound known for its anti-inflammatory properties, but it also plays a significant role in cellular energy production and recovery. MSM helps reduce oxidative stress and inflammation—factors that can impair mitochondrial function. By decreasing inflammation, MSM can enhance mitochondrial activity, improving ATP production. Additionally, MSM supports the synthesis of glutathione, one of the body's primary antioxidants, which is essential for maintaining cellular health and energy metabolism.

A study published in *The Journal of Sports Medicine and Physical Fitness* found that MSM supplementation significantly improved exercise performance and reduced muscle damage in athletes. The reduction of oxidative stress and inflammation led to faster recovery and increased energy levels, supporting the idea that MSM enhances cellular energy production during and after physical activity. MSM's ability to decrease markers of inflammation while boosting antioxidant defense mechanisms, like glutathione, makes it a valuable supplement for enhancing cellular energy production and recovery.

NAC (N-Acetylcysteine)

N-Acetylcysteine (NAC) is a precursor to glutathione, one of the body's most potent antioxidants, playing a critical role in protecting mitochondria from oxidative damage. By increasing glutathione levels, NAC indirectly supports mitochondrial function and energy production. Furthermore, NAC helps reduce oxidative stress and inflammation, both of which can impair cellular energy production.

In a study published in *The American Journal of Clinical Nutrition*, NAC supplementation was found to enhance glutathione levels in cells and protect against oxidative stress-induced damage, especially in individuals exposed to environmental toxins or those with chronic diseases. Moreover, NAC has been shown to improve mitochondrial efficiency, contributing to increased ATP production and better overall cellular energy.

Another study in *The Journal of Molecular Medicine* demonstrated that NAC supplementation improved mitochondrial function and reduced muscle fatigue in patients with chronic obstructive pulmonary disease (COPD), a condition associated with energy metabolism impairments. This study further underscores NAC's role in enhancing energy production by supporting mitochondrial health.

MCT Oil (Medium-Chain Triglycerides)

Medium-Chain Triglycerides (MCTs) are a unique form of dietary fat that is rapidly absorbed and converted into energy by the liver. Unlike long-chain triglycerides, MCTs are broken down quickly and provide an immediate source of fuel, bypassing the typical digestion process. MCT oil has been shown to enhance energy production, support metabolic health, and improve cognitive function, especially when carbohydrates are limited, such as during ketogenic diets.

A study published in *The American Journal of Clinical Nutrition* demonstrated that MCT oil supplementation significantly increased energy expenditure and fat oxidation in individuals following a low-carbohydrate diet. The rapid conversion of MCTs into ketones, an alternative fuel source for the brain and muscles, contributed to enhanced energy production. MCT oil is especially valuable for those seeking a quick energy boost without relying on carbohydrates.

Furthermore, a study in *The Journal of Nutrition* highlighted the role of MCT oil in improving cognitive function in elderly individuals, showing its ability to provide the brain with a fast-acting fuel source. This study also noted that MCT oil supplementation improved mitochondrial efficiency, supporting better energy metabolism at the cellular level.

Melatonin

Melatonin is widely known for its role in regulating sleep cycles, but recent research has uncovered its important role in mitochondrial health and energy production. Melatonin acts as a potent antioxidant that protects mitochondria from oxidative stress, and it has been shown to enhance mitochondrial function by scavenging free radicals and reducing inflammation. Additionally, melatonin plays a role in regulating mitochondrial biogenesis, the process by which new mitochondria are formed in cells.

A study published in *The Journal of Pineal Research* demonstrated that melatonin supplementation increased mitochondrial efficiency and reduced oxidative stress in aging cells. The study highlighted melatonin's role in promoting mitochondrial biogenesis and improving ATP production, which contributes to better energy metabolism. Melatonin's antioxidant properties also protect mitochondria from damage caused by reactive oxygen species (ROS), making it an essential supplement for supporting cellular energy production.

In another study, melatonin was found to protect brain mitochondria from oxidative stress and improve cognitive function, underscoring its importance in maintaining energy production in high-demand tissues like the brain. This makes melatonin not only valuable for sleep regulation but also essential for maintaining mitochondrial health and overall energy production, particularly in aging individuals or those experiencing oxidative stress-related conditions.

Manganese

Manganese is an essential trace mineral that acts as a cofactor for various enzymes involved in energy metabolism and antioxidant defense. One of its most important roles is as a cofactor for the mitochondrial enzyme manganese superoxide dismutase (MnSOD), which protects mitochondria from oxidative stress by neutralizing free radicals. By reducing oxidative damage in mitochondria, manganese supports ATP production and enhances overall energy metabolism.

A study published in *Biological Trace Element Research* found that manganese supplementation increased the activity of MnSOD, leading to reduced oxidative stress and improved mitochondrial function. This research highlighted the importance of manganese in protecting mitochondrial membranes from oxidative damage and supporting efficient energy production.

Additionally, manganese is involved in the metabolism of carbohydrates and fats, contributing to energy generation. Research has shown that manganese deficiency can lead to impaired glucose tolerance and reduced energy metabolism, emphasizing its critical role in maintaining proper cellular energy levels. Ensuring adequate manganese intake is therefore essential for optimizing mitochondrial function and supporting overall cellular energy production.

B Vitamins

B vitamins are a group of water-soluble vitamins that play a crucial role in cellular energy production. Each B vitamin contributes to energy metabolism in different ways. For example:

- Vitamin B1 (Thiamine) is involved in the conversion of carbohydrates into ATP.

- Vitamin B2 (Riboflavin) supports the mitochondrial electron transport chain.
- Vitamin B3 (Niacin) is a precursor to NAD+, which is essential for cellular respiration and ATP production.
- Vitamin B5 (Pantothenic Acid) is a component of coenzyme A, crucial for fatty acid metabolism.
- Vitamin B6 (Pyridoxine) is vital for amino acid metabolism and neurotransmitter synthesis, indirectly supporting energy production.
- Vitamin B9 (Folate) is essential for DNA synthesis and repair, supporting cellular replication and energy metabolism.
- Vitamin B12 (Cobalamin) is important for red blood cell formation and proper nerve function, directly impacting energy levels.

A study published in *The Journal of Nutrition* found that B vitamins play a critical role in energy metabolism by serving as coenzymes for various mitochondrial enzymes involved in ATP production. Supplementing with a B-complex can help maintain optimal energy levels, particularly in individuals with deficiencies due to stress or poor diet.

2. Cell Membrane Health

Cell membranes regulate the flow of substances into and out of cells and play a critical role in cellular communication, protection, and nutrient transport. Damage to these membranes can impair cellular function and lead to inflammation. The following supplements support membrane integrity and enhance cellular resilience:

Phosphatidylcholine

Phosphatidylcholine is a phospholipid and a major component of cell membranes. It helps maintain membrane fluidity and facilitates nutrient transport across the cell membrane. Phosphatidylcholine is also important for liver health and cognitive function. A study published in *Hepatology* showed that phosphatidylcholine supplementation improved liver function and reduced symptoms of fatty liver disease by protecting liver cell membranes. Additionally, research in *The American Journal of Clinical Nutrition* indicated that phosphatidylcholine enhances cognitive function by improving membrane integrity in neurons.

Omega-3 Fatty Acids (EPA and DHA)

Omega-3 fatty acids, particularly EPA and DHA, are essential for the structure and function of cell membranes, especially in the brain and heart. They are incorporated into the phospholipid bilayer, where they improve membrane fluidity and reduce inflammation. A pivotal study in *The American Journal of Clinical Nutrition* found that omega-3 supplementation significantly reduced inflammation and supported cardiovascular health by preserving the integrity of cell membranes. Furthermore, research published in *Neurobiology of Aging* demonstrated that omega-3 fatty acids protect neuronal membranes, reducing the risk of neurodegenerative diseases.

Vitamin E

Vitamin E is a fat-soluble antioxidant that protects cell membranes from oxidative damage by preventing lipid peroxidation—a process that can lead to membrane damage and cell death. Vitamin E is especially important for tissues with high concentrations of polyunsaturated fatty acids, such as the brain and heart. Research published in *Free Radical Biology and Medicine* demonstrated that Vitamin E supplementation protects cell membranes by neutralizing free radicals, thereby reducing lipid peroxidation. This study emphasized Vitamin E's role in preserving membrane integrity and preventing oxidative stress-related damage, which is particularly important for conditions like cardiovascular disease and neurodegeneration.

Methylene Blue

Methylene blue has been studied for its neuroprotective properties, particularly its ability to enhance mitochondrial function and reduce oxidative stress. It also supports cell membrane health by stabilizing the mitochondrial membrane potential, decreasing the production of reactive oxygen species (ROS), and improving mitochondrial efficiency. A study published in *The Journal of Biological Chemistry* found that methylene blue significantly reduced oxidative damage to neuronal cell membranes by decreasing ROS production and enhancing mitochondrial respiration. This makes methylene blue especially useful for preserving cognitive function and preventing membrane damage associated with aging and neurodegenerative diseases.

Zinc

Zinc is crucial for maintaining the structural integrity of cell membranes, particularly in epithelial and immune cells. It aids in membrane repair and protects cells from oxidative damage by acting as a cofactor for antioxidant enzymes. A study in *Nutrients* reported that zinc supplementation improved the integrity of the gut barrier by supporting epithelial cell membranes, which helps prevent inflammation and maintains cellular homeostasis. Zinc's role in membrane repair makes it essential for immune function and overall cellular health.

Copper

Copper plays a critical role in maintaining cell membrane integrity by acting as a cofactor for superoxide dismutase (SOD), an antioxidant enzyme that protects against oxidative stress. Copper is also necessary for collagen production, which supports the structural stability of cell membranes and surrounding tissues. A study published in *BioMetals* found that copper deficiency impairs the body's ability to protect cell membranes from oxidative damage, leading to increased lipid peroxidation. Supplementing with copper helps prevent this oxidative stress and supports the long-term health of tissues like the skin, lungs, and blood vessels.

Curcumin

Curcumin, the active compound in turmeric, is widely recognized for its potent anti-inflammatory and antioxidant properties. It plays a crucial role in maintaining cell membrane integrity by neutralizing free radicals and reducing inflammation—both of which can damage cell membranes. Curcumin has been shown to stabilize the lipid bilayer of membranes, ensuring their fluidity and functionality.

A study published in *Biochimica et Biophysica Acta (BBA) - Biomembranes* revealed that curcumin helps maintain membrane integrity by directly interacting with membrane lipids, thereby protecting them from oxidative stress-induced damage. The study demonstrated that curcumin's antioxidant activity helps stabilize cell membranes, particularly in tissues prone to inflammation, such as the liver and cardiovascular system.

Additionally, curcumin has been found to enhance the membrane's response to external stimuli, supporting better cell signaling and function. This is particularly beneficial in preventing inflammatory diseases where membrane integrity is compromised. Curcumin's ability to reduce chronic inflammation and oxidative stress makes it an essential supplement for maintaining the health and function of cell membranes, especially in individuals prone to chronic conditions such as arthritis or cardiovascular disorders.

Pterostilbene

Pterostilbene is a natural compound closely related to resveratrol, primarily found in blueberries and grapes. Like resveratrol, pterostilbene has powerful antioxidant properties that protect cell membranes from oxidative damage. It has been shown to enhance membrane fluidity and stability, particularly in neurons and cardiovascular cells, where oxidative stress can lead to inflammation and cell death.

A study published in *Oxidative Medicine and Cellular Longevity* found that pterostilbene improved the structural integrity of cell membranes by reducing lipid peroxidation, a process that damages membrane phospholipids. The study highlighted that pterostilbene's potent antioxidant activity not only prevents oxidative damage but also promotes cell membrane longevity.

In another study, pterostilbene was shown to improve cognitive function by protecting neuronal membranes from oxidative stress. This is especially significant in preventing neurodegenerative conditions, such as Alzheimer's disease, where membrane damage plays a crucial role in disease progression. The study concluded that regular supplementation with pterostilbene could help maintain membrane fluidity and functionality, particularly in aging populations.

Vitamin C

Vitamin C is well-known for its antioxidant properties but also plays a crucial role in maintaining the stability and integrity of cell membranes. It is essential for the synthesis of collagen, a structural protein that supports cell membrane stability, particularly in the skin, blood vessels, and connective tissues. Additionally, Vitamin C helps protect membranes from oxidative stress by neutralizing free radicals.

Research published in *The American Journal of Clinical Nutrition* demonstrated that Vitamin C supplementation significantly reduced oxidative damage to cell membranes, particularly in individuals with higher oxidative stress levels due to smoking or exposure to environmental pollutants. The study concluded that Vitamin C enhances the structural stability of membranes by supporting collagen synthesis and protecting against free radical damage.

Moreover, Vitamin C's role in maintaining membrane stability is essential for wound healing and skin health. Another study found that Vitamin C supplementation improved skin barrier function by supporting membrane integrity, making it a critical supplement for maintaining healthy, resilient tissues.

Resveratrol is a polyphenol found in grapes, red wine, and berries, known for its potent antioxidant properties. It supports cell membrane health by protecting lipids in the membrane from oxidative damage and improving overall membrane fluidity. Resveratrol also activates SIRT1, a protein associated with longevity, and promotes mitochondrial function, thereby supporting both membrane stability and energy production.

A study published in *Nature* demonstrated that resveratrol supplementation improved mitochondrial function and protected cell membranes from lipid peroxidation in animal models. The study also found that resveratrol enhances the membrane's ability to resist oxidative stress, which is crucial for preventing age-related membrane damage.

3. Cellular Terrain Health

Maintaining a healthy cellular terrain—the internal environment of cells—is essential for optimal immune response, nutrient absorption, detoxification, and the prevention of chronic diseases. The following supplements contribute significantly to optimizing this internal environment, enhancing cellular function, and promoting long-term well-being:

Sodium butyrate not only enhances gut health but also reduces inflammation throughout the body, promoting a balanced immune response. Studies have shown that sodium butyrate supplementation improves gut barrier function, helping to prevent the translocation of harmful bacteria and toxins from the gut into the bloodstream, thereby reducing systemic inflammation.

A study published in *Gut* found that sodium butyrate enhanced intestinal barrier function and reduced inflammation in patients with inflammatory bowel disease (IBD). These results suggest that sodium butyrate may be a key supplement for maintaining gut health and reducing chronic inflammation, which in turn supports the cellular terrain.

Pre- and Probiotics

Probiotics are live bacteria that promote a healthy gut microbiome, while prebiotics are non-digestible fibers that nourish these beneficial bacteria. Together, they support digestion, nutrient absorption, and immune function. A balanced gut microbiome plays a crucial role in maintaining cellular terrain by ensuring proper nutrient absorption, reducing inflammation, and supporting detoxification.

Clinical trials have demonstrated that probiotic supplementation can improve gut health by restoring the balance of beneficial bacteria, enhancing immune response, and alleviating symptoms of gastrointestinal disorders. For instance, a study published in *The British Journal of Nutrition* found that probiotics significantly reduced markers of inflammation and improved gut barrier integrity in patients with irritable bowel syndrome (IBS).

Prebiotics, such as inulin and fructooligosaccharides, further support this balance by feeding beneficial bacteria and promoting their growth. By improving the gut microbiome, pre- and probiotics help optimize nutrient absorption and reduce systemic inflammation, thereby promoting a healthy cellular environment.

Selenium

Selenium is an essential trace mineral that works in synergy with glutathione to enhance antioxidant defenses and reduce oxidative stress. It is also critical for immune function and thyroid health. Deficiency in selenium is linked to an increased risk of chronic diseases. A study published in *The Lancet* demonstrated that selenium supplementation enhanced immune function, reduced oxidative stress, and lowered the risk of certain cancers, particularly in selenium-deficient populations. Selenium's role in supporting antioxidant activity and immune health makes it essential for maintaining a healthy cellular terrain and protecting against disease.

Magnesium

Magnesium is essential not only for energy production but also for regulating inflammation and supporting detoxification processes. Magnesium deficiency has been linked to increased oxidative stress and inflammation, which can compromise cellular health. A study published in *The Journal of Inflammation Research* found that magnesium supplementation significantly reduced markers of chronic inflammation in individuals with low magnesium levels. By improving antioxidant capacity and reducing inflammation, magnesium supports a balanced cellular terrain, contributing to overall health and well-being.

Iron

Iron is vital for oxygen transport and cellular respiration, playing a key role in energy metabolism. It is a central component of hemoglobin, which carries oxygen from the lungs to tissues throughout the body, ensuring that cells have sufficient oxygen to produce ATP. A study published in *The American Journal of Clinical Nutrition* demonstrated that iron supplementation improved energy metabolism and reduced symptoms of fatigue in individuals with iron deficiency anemia. Maintaining adequate iron levels ensures that cells receive enough oxygen to function efficiently, which is critical for maintaining a healthy cellular environment.

Curcumin

Curcumin, the active compound in turmeric, is known for its powerful anti-inflammatory and antioxidant properties. It supports cellular health by reducing oxidative stress and inflammation—both key contributors to chronic diseases. Curcumin also enhances detoxification by promoting the activity of liver enzymes involved in the removal of toxins from the body. A study published in *The Journal of Clinical Immunology* demonstrated that curcumin supplementation reduced inflammation and oxidative stress in patients with rheumatoid arthritis, suggesting its potential for supporting cellular terrain health by reducing systemic inflammation.

Berberine is a plant compound with anti-inflammatory, antimicrobial, and blood sugar-lowering properties. It supports cellular terrain health by improving glucose metabolism, reducing inflammation, and supporting gut health. Berberine activates AMPK (adenosine monophosphate-activated protein kinase), a key energy-sensing enzyme, making it particularly effective in regulating metabolism and improving insulin sensitivity.

A study published in *Metabolism: Clinical and Experimental* showed that berberine supplementation improved insulin sensitivity and reduced markers of inflammation in patients with type 2 diabetes. Berberine's impact on metabolism and inflammation makes it a valuable supplement for maintaining cellular health, especially in individuals with metabolic syndrome.

Quercetin is a flavonoid with potent antioxidant and anti-inflammatory properties. It helps protect cells from oxidative damage and supports immune function by modulating inflammatory pathways. Quercetin has also been shown to improve cardiovascular health by reducing oxidative stress in blood vessels, thereby protecting endothelial cells.

A study published in *The American Journal of Clinical Nutrition* found that quercetin supplementation significantly reduced oxidative stress and improved blood vessel function in patients with cardiovascular disease. By reducing oxidative stress and inflammation, quercetin supports the cellular terrain and helps protect against chronic diseases.

Ashwagandha is an adaptogen, meaning it helps the body adapt to stress by modulating the stress response and supporting adrenal health. It has been shown to reduce cortisol levels, improve immune function, and enhance overall resilience to stress, which can have a profound impact on cellular health. A study published in *The Journal of Clinical Psychology* found that ashwagandha supplementation reduced stress and anxiety in individuals with chronic stress, suggesting that it supports the cellular terrain by improving the body's ability to cope with both physical and emotional stress.

EGCG (Epigallocatechin Gallate)

Epigallocatechin gallate (EGCG), the active component in green tea, is a powerful antioxidant that protects cells from oxidative damage and supports overall cellular health. Research has shown that EGCG enhances detoxification by promoting liver function and reducing inflammation. Additionally, EGCG supports mitochondrial function and improves fat metabolism, contributing to better energy production and weight management.

A study published in *The Journal of Nutritional Biochemistry* demonstrated that EGCG supplementation reduced markers of oxidative stress and inflammation in individuals with cardiovascular risk factors. The study concluded that EGCG's potent antioxidant properties help protect cells from free radical damage and support overall cellular health. By reducing oxidative stress and enhancing detoxification, EGCG plays a significant role in maintaining a healthy cellular environment, particularly for individuals at risk of cardiovascular disease, obesity, or metabolic disorders.

Carbon 60 (C60) is a powerful antioxidant composed of 60 carbon atoms arranged in a spherical structure. Known for its ability to neutralize free radicals, C60 protects cells from oxidative damage, which can accelerate aging and contribute to chronic diseases. C60 has been shown to improve mitochondrial function by increasing ATP production and reducing oxidative stress, making it an effective supplement for cellular repair and longevity.

A study published in *Biomaterials Science* demonstrated that C60 supplementation extended the lifespan of mice by protecting cells from oxidative damage and improving mitochondrial function. The study also highlighted C60's potential anti-aging properties, making it a promising supplement for maintaining a healthy cellular environment and promoting long-term vitality. By enhancing mitochondrial function and reducing oxidative stress, C60 helps protect cells from the damage associated with aging, inflammation, and chronic diseases.

The supplements discussed in this section—each supported by scientific studies—offer various benefits for cellular health. By optimizing cellular energy production, maintaining cell membrane health, and improving the cellular environment, these supplements contribute to overall health and longevity. Integrating these supplements into a daily routine, alongside a balanced diet and healthy lifestyle, provides targeted support for energy metabolism, immune function, detoxification, and protection against oxidative stress and inflammation. Nourishing the body at a cellular level can enhance resilience to stress, reduce the risk of chronic diseases, and promote long-term vitality.

Supplementation Strategies: Best Practices for Integrating Supplements into a Daily Routine

While supplements can effectively support cellular health, it's important to approach supplementation with a clear strategy to ensure optimal results. Here are some best practices for incorporating supplements into your daily routine:

Personalize Your Supplement Plan

Not all supplements are necessary for everyone. The specific supplements you need will depend on factors such as age, diet, lifestyle, and health goals. Before starting any supplement regimen, it's a good idea to consult with a healthcare professional or nutritionist who can help identify any nutritional gaps or deficiencies. Blood tests and other assessments can offer valuable insights into which nutrients your body may need. With a clearer understanding of your unique needs, you can create a personalized supplement plan that targets specific areas like mitochondrial function, cognitive performance, or immune support.

Prioritize Quality Over Quantity

The quality of the supplements you choose is just as important as the nutrients themselves. Many low-cost supplements contain fillers, additives, and synthetic ingredients that can reduce effectiveness or even cause harm. Look for high-quality supplements from reputable brands that use third-party testing to verify purity and potency. Choose supplements made from natural, bioavailable forms of nutrients that your body can easily absorb. For example, opt for ubiquinol (the active form of CoQ10) over ubiquinone, or choose liposomal formulations of nutrients like vitamin C and glutathione for enhanced absorption.

Incorporate Supplements into Your Routine

Consistency is key when it comes to supplementation. Make supplements part of your daily routine by setting reminders, keeping them in a visible place, or integrating them into meals or morning/evening rituals. Some supplements, like CoQ10 and fat-soluble vitamins (A, D, E, and K), are better absorbed when taken with food, especially meals containing healthy fats. Others, such as methylene blue or taurine, can be taken at any time of day.

Monitor Progress and Adjust as Needed

Track how your body responds to supplements and adjust as necessary. Keep a journal or log to note any improvements in energy levels, cognitive function, or overall well-being. Some supplements, like taurine or CoQ10, may produce noticeable effects within a few weeks, while others, like C60 or phosphatidylcholine, may take longer to show results. If you experience side effects or if a supplement doesn't seem effective, consider adjusting the dosage or trying a different form. Regular check-ins with your healthcare provider can help ensure your supplement plan remains aligned with your health goals.

Supplements work best when combined with a healthy diet, regular exercise, and stress management. Focus on a nutrient-dense, anti-inflammatory diet rich in fruits, vegetables, healthy fats, and lean proteins to support overall health and provide the raw materials your cells need to thrive. Regular physical activity stimulates mitochondrial function and promotes cellular repair. Practices such as mindfulness, meditation, and getting adequate sleep are also essential for reducing stress and supporting the body's natural healing processes.

Conclusion

Supplements play a crucial role in supporting and enhancing cellular health by filling nutritional gaps, optimizing energy production, maintaining cell membrane integrity, and improving the internal cellular environment. As we navigate the complexities of modern life, where dietary choices may not always provide all the nutrients our bodies need, these supplements can be valuable allies in promoting resilience, vitality, and overall well-being.

By incorporating a carefully selected range of supplements—such as CoQ10 for energy production, omega-3 fatty acids for membrane health, and probiotics for gut health—individuals can bolster cellular function and mitigate the effects of oxidative stress and inflammation. However, it is essential to personalize supplementation plans, prioritize high-quality products, and integrate these practices into a holistic lifestyle that includes a balanced diet, regular exercise, and effective stress management.

In the next chapter, *Innovative Therapies for Cellular Health*, we will explore cutting-edge approaches and therapies that further enhance cellular function and support the body's innate healing abilities. From emerging technologies to novel treatment methods, this chapter will highlight how innovative therapies are revolutionizing our understanding of cellular health and paving the way for improved wellness and longevity.

CHAPTER FOURTEEN

Therapies for Cellular Health

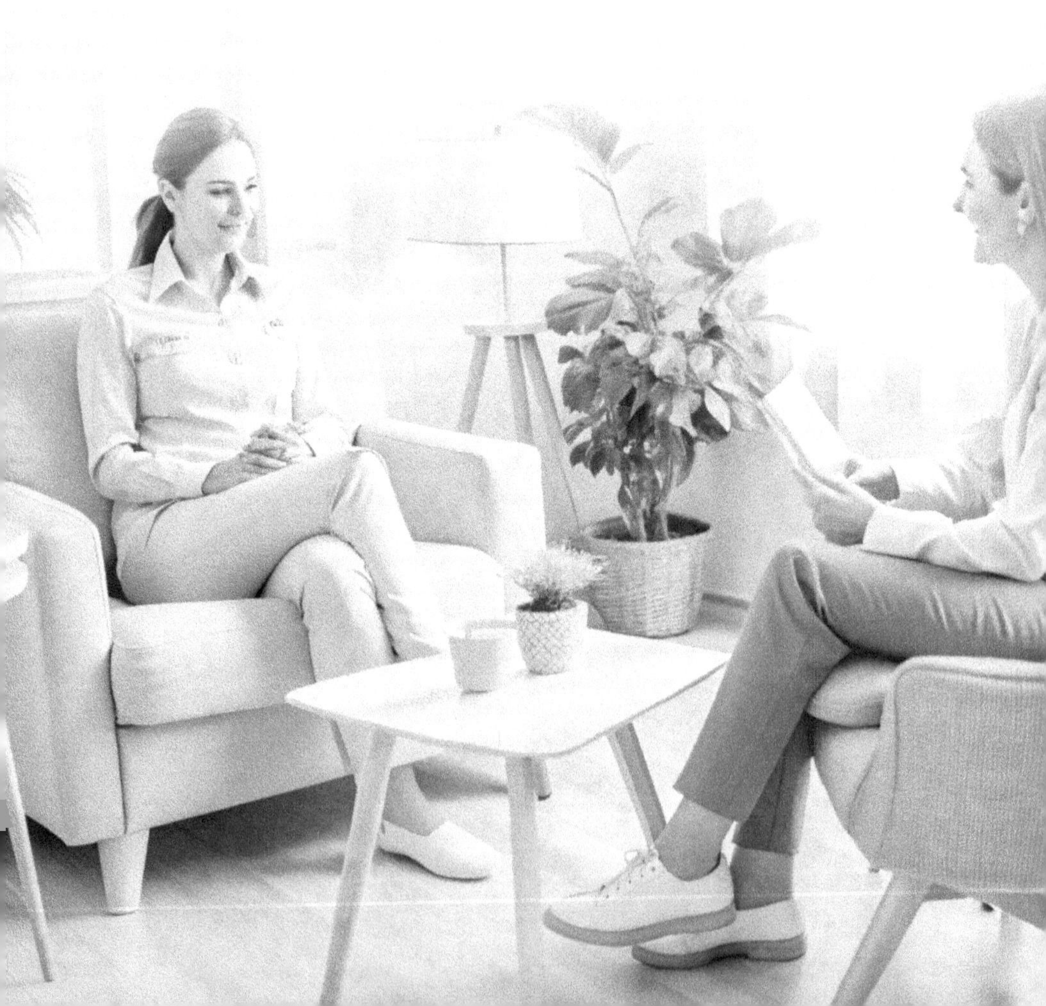

"Healing is a matter of time, but it is sometimes also a matter of opportunity."
—Hippocrates

Hippocrates' timeless wisdom emphasizes the body's inherent ability to heal, alongside the importance of timely interventions that can enhance this process. As our understanding of cellular biology continues to grow, a range of innovative therapies has emerged, aimed at optimizing cellular function, repairing damage, and restoring balance. These advanced treatments offer solutions for health challenges that may not respond fully to conventional methods, serving as powerful complements to traditional practices. In this chapter, we will explore various therapies that support cellular health, including Bioenergetics, ozone sauna therapy, Pulsed Electromagnetic Field (PEMF) therapy, red light/near-infrared (NIR) therapy, and intravenous (IV) nutritional therapy. We will explain how these therapies work at the cellular level, what individuals might experience, and why they are crucial for enhancing overall vitality.

Bioenergetics

Bioenergetics operates on the principle that all living organisms are governed by energy fields that influence health. By addressing imbalances in these energy fields, bioenergetic therapies aim to restore harmony within the body, thus promoting healing. Techniques such as energy healing, sound therapy, and light therapy are used to enhance the body's energy flow and optimize cellular function.

One specific approach within bioenergetics is NES Health, which combines insights from quantum physics with traditional medicine to assess and restore the body's energy field. Using advanced technology, NES Health identifies blockages in energy flow and recommends remedies to facilitate healing. By addressing these disruptions, NES Health promotes better nutrient absorption, improved cellular repair, and enhanced detoxification.

The physiological benefits of bioenergetic therapies are profound. They support mitochondrial function—the powerhouses of our cells responsible for energy production—by enhancing ATP synthesis and promoting cellular communication. When energy flows freely through the body, cellular processes can function optimally, leading to improved metabolism, greater resilience to stress, and enhanced immune function. Research indicates that energy healing modalities can lower stress hormones like cortisol, which are linked to inflammation and cellular aging. By reducing these stress responses, bioenergetics helps cultivate a balanced cellular environment conducive to repair and regeneration.

Our bodies are made of energy, and when our energy levels become depleted, we may experience symptoms ranging from fatigue to more severe health issues. Continued depletion can lead to diseases and, ultimately, cell death. Therefore, supporting our energy levels and ensuring they remain adequate is key to maintaining cellular vitality.

Ozone Sauna Therapy

Ozone sauna therapy combines the benefits of ozone gas (O_3) with the detoxifying effects of heat to stimulate cellular healing. By introducing ozone into the body, this therapy enhances oxygen availability and promotes the breakdown of harmful pathogens, making it effective for various health challenges, including infections, autoimmune conditions, and chronic inflammation.

The mechanism of ozone therapy lies in its ability to increase oxygen levels in tissues and stimulate the production of antioxidant enzymes, such as superoxide dismutase (SOD). These enzymes are crucial for neutralizing free radicals and mitigating oxidative stress within cells. A study published in *The Journal of Clinical Investigation* demonstrated that ozone therapy significantly increases SOD levels, enhancing the body's antioxidant defenses and protecting cells from oxidative damage.

Ozone therapy also induces a hyperthermic effect due to the sauna environment, promoting detoxification through sweating and improving circulation. This combination not only enhances oxygen delivery to tissues but also stimulates cellular repair processes. Patients undergoing ozone sauna therapy often report increased energy levels, improved immune response, and a reduction in symptoms related to chronic conditions.

The ability of ozone to enhance mitochondrial function further underscores its role in promoting cellular health. Improved oxygen utilization and reduced oxidative stress support cellular integrity, allowing for optimal functionality and resilience against environmental toxins. Ozone sauna therapy, therefore, represents a multifaceted approach to cellular health that encompasses detoxification, enhanced energy production, and immune support.

Pulsed Electromagnetic Field (PEMF) Therapy

PEMF therapy is a non-invasive treatment that uses low-frequency electromagnetic pulses to stimulate and repair cells at a cellular level. This therapy is based on the principle that all living organisms are composed of electromagnetic fields, which significantly influence cellular function and communication.

The primary mechanism of PEMF therapy is its ability to enhance mitochondrial function, which is critical for energy production. Research indicates that PEMF therapy can significantly increase ATP production—some studies report increases of up to 500%. For instance, a study published in *Electromagnetic Biology and Medicine* highlighted that PEMF therapy enhances mitochondrial bioenergetics, improving cellular metabolism and facilitating tissue regeneration.

Additionally, PEMF therapy improves circulation by stimulating the production of nitric oxide, a vasodilator that enhances blood flow to tissues. This increase in circulation allows for better oxygen and nutrient delivery, both of which are vital for cellular repair and regeneration. According to research published in *The Journal of Orthopaedic Research*, PEMF therapy has been shown to accelerate healing in non-union bone fractures and reduce postoperative pain and swelling.

At the cellular level, PEMF therapy supports the body's natural repair processes by enhancing ATP production, improving nutrient delivery, and facilitating waste removal. Patients often experience reduced inflammation, improved mobility, and faster recovery times, demonstrating the powerful impact of this therapy on cellular health.

Red Light/Near-Infrared (NIR) Therapy

Red light and near-infrared (NIR) therapy utilizes specific wavelengths of light to penetrate tissues and stimulate cellular processes, promoting healing and energy production. This therapy is based on the principle that light can induce biological effects on living organisms, particularly at the cellular level.

The primary mechanism of action involves the stimulation of mitochondrial function through the absorption of light energy by photoreceptors in the mitochondria. This process enhances ATP production, providing the energy necessary for cellular repair and regeneration. A study published in *Photomedicine and Laser Surgery* found that red light therapy significantly improved mitochondrial function, leading to enhanced energy metabolism and increased cellular repair.

Additionally, red light therapy has been shown to reduce inflammation and oxidative stress. Research indicates that exposure to red light can increase the production of antioxidant enzymes, which further protect cells from damage. By promoting blood flow and oxygen delivery to tissues, red light therapy facilitates faster healing and recovery.

At the cellular level, red light and NIR therapy improve mitochondrial efficiency and support cellular regeneration. By increasing the energy available to cells, this therapy aids in various healing processes, including tissue repair and inflammation reduction. Patients with chronic pain, muscle soreness, and joint issues often find relief through red light therapy, which promotes healing at the cellular level and enhances overall vitality.

Intravenous (IV) Nutritional Therapy

Intravenous (IV) nutritional therapy delivers essential vitamins, minerals, and amino acids directly into the bloodstream, bypassing the digestive system for immediate absorption. This method is particularly advantageous for individuals who are nutrient-deficient or have increased nutrient needs due to illness, malabsorption, or physical stress.

The mechanism of action for IV nutritional therapy allows for the direct infusion of bioavailable nutrients, which can be immediately utilized by cells. This direct delivery method is critical for patients with malabsorption issues, ensuring that essential nutrients reach their targets without digestive barriers. Common nutrients administered via IV include vitamin C, B vitamins, magnesium, and glutathione—all of which support mitochondrial function, reduce oxidative stress, and promote cellular repair.

For instance, a study published in *Nutrients* showed that IV vitamin C significantly reduces oxidative stress by increasing the availability of antioxidants and supporting mitochondrial function. Vitamin C also plays a role in collagen synthesis, vital for maintaining healthy connective tissues and cellular structures. Similarly, IV magnesium has been shown to improve cardiovascular health and enhance energy production by aiding ATP synthesis. Furthermore, IV glutathione supports detoxification and immune function by helping the liver process toxins and repair damaged tissues.

IV nutritional therapy provides rapid, targeted nutrient support, promoting energy production, cellular repair, and overall well-being. This therapy is especially beneficial for individuals recovering from surgery, those with nutrient deficiencies, or athletes needing enhanced recovery and performance. Importantly, IV nutritional therapy can support cellular energy, membrane integrity, and the cellular terrain, addressing multiple facets of cellular health.

Comprehensive Benefits of Innovative Therapies

All the therapies discussed—Bioenergetics, ozone sauna therapy, PEMF therapy, red light/NIR therapy, and IV nutritional therapy—are effective in supporting cellular health. They enhance cellular ATP production, improve cell membrane health, and optimize the cellular terrain, which is the internal environment that supports cellular function.

These therapies facilitate detoxification and engage in what can be described as "cellular exercise," where cells undergo processes that enhance their resilience and vitality. For example, ozone therapy promotes oxygen utilization and detoxification, while PEMF therapy enhances mitochondrial function, leading to increased ATP production. Red light therapy aids in reducing oxidative stress and promoting cellular repair, and IV nutritional therapy ensures the necessary nutrients are available for optimal cellular function.

When combined, these therapies create a powerful synergistic effect that enhances energy production, improves cellular communication, and optimizes detoxification processes. This multifaceted approach is particularly beneficial for individuals facing chronic health challenges, as it supports the body's innate healing abilities and promotes long-term health and well-being.

When to Consider These Therapies

These advanced therapies are particularly useful for individuals dealing with chronic or recurrent health issues, poor nutrient absorption, post-surgery recovery, or those seeking to enhance athletic performance. They can also be valuable for preventing disease by addressing oxidative stress and inflammation before they escalate into more serious health concerns. Consulting with a healthcare professional can help determine the most suitable therapies based on individual health needs and goals, unlocking the potential for accelerated healing and enhanced vitality.

By understanding how these therapies work and when they may be appropriate, you can make informed decisions about incorporating them into your health regimen. This knowledge empowers you to unlock the benefits of enhanced cellular repair, energy production, and overall vitality.

Conclusion

Innovative therapies such as Bioenergetics, ozone sauna therapy, PEMF therapy, red light/NIR therapy, and IV nutritional therapy represent powerful tools for optimizing cellular health. Each of these therapies addresses the fundamental aspects of cellular function, from enhancing energy production to improving detoxification and reducing oxidative stress. As we navigate a world filled with environmental stressors and health challenges, integrating these therapies into our wellness plans can significantly enhance our overall vitality and resilience. The combined benefits of these treatments work synergistically to create an environment that supports optimal cellular health, making them invaluable for anyone looking to elevate their well-being.

As we move into the next chapter, *"Creating a Cellular Wellness Plan,"* we will explore how to effectively integrate these therapies into a comprehensive health strategy tailored to individual needs, ensuring that the journey to cellular vitality is both sustainable and effective.

CHAPTER FIFTEEN

Creating a Cellular Wellness Plan

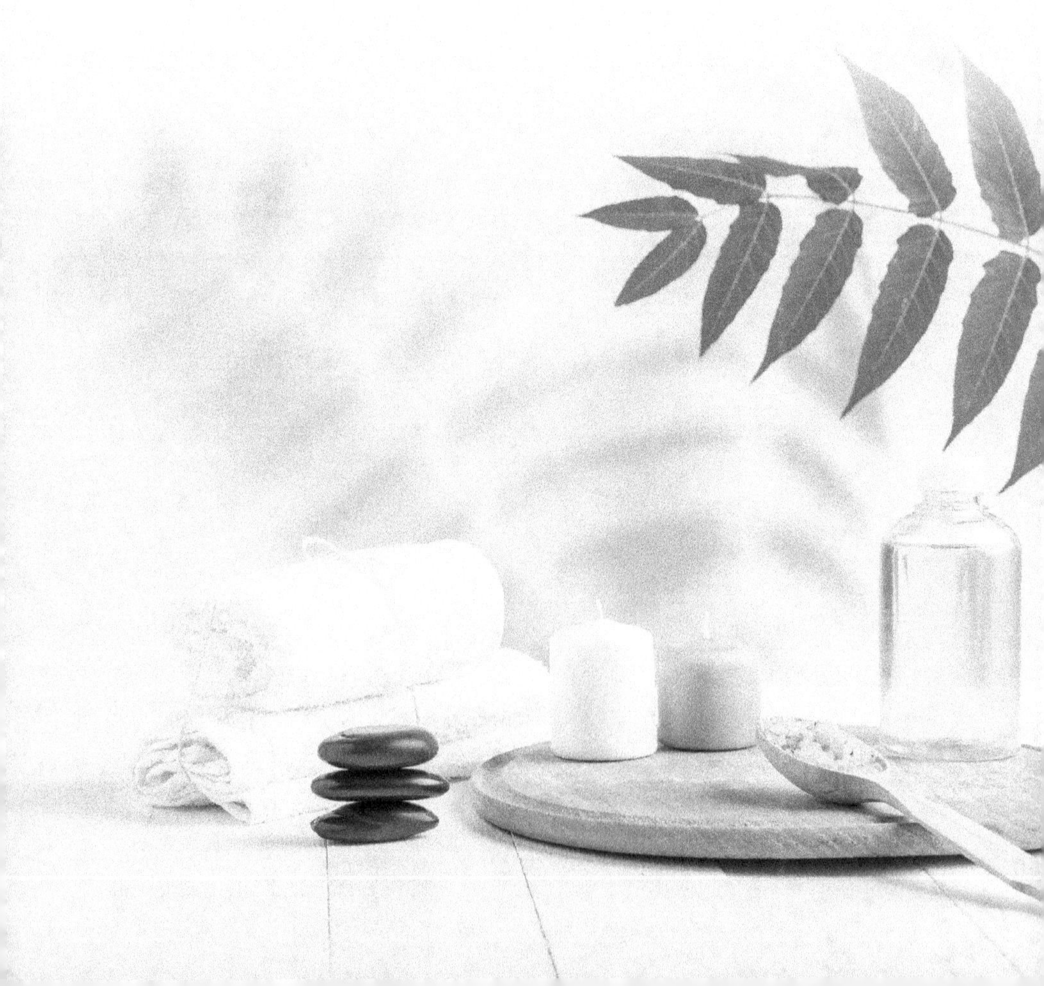

"An ounce of prevention is worth a pound of cure." —Benjamin Franklin

Benjamin Franklin's timeless words, "An ounce of prevention is worth a pound of cure," remind us that taking proactive steps to care for our health today can help prevent more serious issues down the road. This is particularly true when it comes to cellular health. By addressing the factors that impact our cells—such as nutrition, stress, toxins, and mitochondrial function—we can support our body's ability to repair and regenerate itself, maintain energy levels, and reduce the risk of chronic disease. In this chapter, we'll discuss how to create a personalized cellular wellness plan that focuses on prevention and optimization, incorporating diet, lifestyle changes, supplements, and therapies. We'll also explore tools and strategies for tracking your progress and monitoring improvements in cellular health.

How to Create a Personalized Cellular Wellness Plan

To create a personalized cellular wellness plan, take a holistic approach by considering both your current health status and long-term goals. Below is a step-by-step guide to building a comprehensive plan that addresses all aspects of cellular health:

Assess Your Current Health Status

Before developing your plan, assess your current health, including any underlying conditions, nutrient deficiencies, or lifestyle factors that may be contributing to cellular dysfunction. Consider these steps:

- **Health History Review**: Reflect on any existing health conditions, such as chronic fatigue, digestive issues, inflammation, or metabolic disorders. These can provide insight into areas where cellular function may need support.
- **Blood Tests and Assessments**: Work with a healthcare professional to order blood tests that evaluate key markers of cellular health, such as mitochondrial function, oxidative stress, inflammation, and nutrient levels (e.g., CoQ10, glutathione, vitamins, minerals). This data will help identify any deficiencies or imbalances.
- **Lifestyle Evaluation**: Assess your daily habits, including diet, exercise, sleep patterns, and stress levels. Identifying areas where improvements can be made will provide a starting point for your wellness plan.

For example, if blood tests reveal low CoQ10 levels and high oxidative stress, your plan may include supplements targeting mitochondrial health and antioxidant support, along with dietary changes to reduce inflammation.

Set Specific Health Goals

Having clear, measurable health goals will help guide your plan and allow you to track your progress over time. These goals can include anything from improving energy levels and reducing inflammation to enhancing cognitive function or optimizing athletic performance.

Sample Goals:
- Increase energy levels by 20% within three months.
- Improve sleep quality by reducing nighttime awakenings from five to two per night.

- Reduce markers of inflammation (e.g., CRP levels) by 50% over six months.
- Enhance recovery time after exercise or injury by supporting mitochondrial function.

Design a Nutrient-Dense, Anti-Inflammatory Diet

Nutrition is the cornerstone of cellular health. A diet rich in whole, nutrient-dense foods provides your cells with the fuel they need for repair, energy production, and detoxification. Key components of a cellular wellness diet include:

- **Antioxidant-Rich Foods**: To protect cells from oxidative damage, include a variety of antioxidant-rich foods, such as berries, leafy greens, dark chocolate, nuts, seeds, and green tea.
- **Healthy Fats**: Fats are essential for maintaining the structure of cell membranes and supporting brain and mitochondrial health. Include omega-3 fatty acids from fatty fish, flaxseeds, and walnuts, as well as monounsaturated fats from avocados and olive oil.
- **High-Quality Proteins**: Protein is necessary for repairing and regenerating tissues. Focus on clean sources of protein, such as grass-fed beef, wild-caught fish, organic poultry, and plant-based proteins like lentils, quinoa, and hemp seeds.
- **Anti-Inflammatory Foods**: To reduce inflammation, include anti-inflammatory foods such as turmeric, ginger, garlic, green leafy vegetables, and cruciferous vegetables (e.g., broccoli, cauliflower).

- **Hydration:** Stay hydrated by drinking plenty of water throughout the day. Proper hydration supports cellular function, aids in detoxification, and helps maintain energy levels.

Example:

A daily meal plan might include a smoothie with spinach, blueberries, flaxseeds, and almond butter for breakfast; a salad with wild salmon, avocado, and lemon-olive oil dressing for lunch; and roasted vegetables with grass-fed beef for dinner.

Incorporate Lifestyle Changes

Your lifestyle habits have a significant impact on cellular health. Chronic stress, poor sleep, and lack of physical activity can all contribute to cellular dysfunction. By making the following lifestyle changes, you can support your cells:

- **Reduce Stress:** Chronic stress elevates cortisol levels, which can impair cellular repair and increase inflammation. Incorporate stress-reduction practices such as meditation, deep breathing exercises, yoga, or spending time in nature to help lower stress and promote relaxation.
- **Prioritize Sleep:** Sleep is essential for cellular repair and regeneration. Aim for 7–9 hours of quality sleep each night and create a calming bedtime routine that supports relaxation. This might include avoiding screens before bed, using blackout curtains, or practicing mindfulness.
- **Move Regularly:** Regular exercise enhances mitochondrial function, improves circulation, and promotes detoxification. Incorporate a mix of

cardiovascular exercise, strength training, and flexibility work (e.g., yoga or Pilates) into your routine.

- **Detoxification Support**: Support your body's natural detoxification processes by incorporating practices such as dry brushing, saunas, and Epsom salt baths, all of which help remove toxins and reduce the burden on your cells.

Example:

A daily cellular wellness routine might include 10 minutes of meditation in the morning, a 30-minute walk after lunch, and 20 minutes of stretching or yoga before bed.

Add Targeted Supplements

Once you've addressed diet and lifestyle changes, supplements can provide additional support for cellular health. Some key supplements to consider include:

- **Magnesium**: Essential for ATP production, mitochondrial function, and overall cellular health.
- **CoQ10**: Supports mitochondrial function and energy production, especially for individuals with low CoQ10 levels.
- **Taurine**: Protects against oxidative stress and supports cellular detoxification.
- **Phosphatidylcholine**: Maintains the integrity of cell membranes and supports liver and brain health.

- **Glutathione**: The body's master antioxidant, which helps neutralize free radicals and supports detoxification.
- **Omega-3 Fatty Acids**: Reduce inflammation and support cardiovascular and brain health.
- **B Vitamins**: Crucial for mitochondrial function and energy metabolism, supporting the conversion of food into usable energy.
- **Vitamin D**: Enhances immune function, reduces inflammation, and supports overall cellular health. Vitamin D3 should be taken with K2 to help calcium stay in the bones rather than forming plaque in the arteries.

Example:

If you're focusing on energy production and mitochondrial health, you might include a supplement stack with CoQ10, alpha-lipoic acid, and acetyl-L-carnitine.

Explore Innovative Therapies

As part of a comprehensive wellness plan, incorporating innovative therapies such as Bioenergetics, PEMF (Pulsed Electromagnetic Field) therapy, ozone therapy, and IV nutrition can significantly enhance cellular health and accelerate recovery. These therapies target underlying cellular dysfunction, improve nutrient absorption, and promote faster healing. For individuals with chronic conditions like autoimmune disorders, chronic pain, or inflammation, PEMF therapy can stimulate tissue regeneration and reduce inflammation. In cases of poor nutrient absorption, IV nutrition ensures essential vitamins and minerals are delivered directly to the bloodstream, bypassing digestive issues.

For post-surgical recovery or trauma, PEMF and IV nutrition therapies can enhance circulation, reduce oxidative stress, and speed tissue repair. Additionally, ozone therapy may boost immune function and reduce the risk of infection, especially in patients with weakened immune systems or chronic infections. For athletes or highly active individuals, these therapies can optimize performance, enhance muscle recovery, and prevent injury.

Together, these therapies offer a holistic, integrative approach to support long-term health, healing, and overall well-being. By customizing the plan to meet each patient's specific needs and goals, these treatments ensure personalized care that promotes optimal cellular health.

Tracking Your Progress: Tools and Tips for Monitoring Improvements in Cellular Health

Tracking your progress is an essential part of any wellness plan. It allows you to see what's working, make necessary adjustments, and stay motivated as you work toward your health goals. Below are some effective tools and strategies for monitoring improvements in your cellular health over time:

1. Regular Blood Testing

One of the most reliable ways to track cellular health is through regular blood testing. Tests that measure inflammation (e.g., CRP levels), oxidative stress markers, mitochondrial function, and nutrient levels can provide valuable insights into how well your plan is working. Depending on your goals, you may want to test these markers every 3–6 months. For example, if reducing inflammation is one of your objectives, track your CRP levels and note any reductions after implementing your cellular wellness plan.

2. Energy and Mood Tracking

Keep a journal or use a health app to track your daily energy levels, mood, and cognitive function. Over time, you should notice improvements as your cellular function improves. Be sure to note how you feel after incorporating specific supplements, lifestyle changes, or therapies. You can track your energy on a scale from 1–10 each day, paying attention to any patterns or improvements as you adjust your routine.

3. Fitness and Recovery Metrics

If your goal is to improve physical performance or recovery, use fitness tracking devices to monitor areas such as endurance, strength, heart rate variability (HRV), and recovery time. HRV, in particular, is a useful marker of cellular resilience and autonomic nervous system balance. You can use a fitness tracker or app to monitor your HRV before and after implementing stress-reduction techniques or starting a mitochondrial support supplement regimen.

4. Sleep Quality Monitoring

If improving sleep is one of your health goals, use sleep-tracking tools (such as wearable devices or apps) to monitor metrics like total sleep time, sleep efficiency, and the duration of deep or REM sleep. Improved sleep quality is a key indicator that your body is undergoing proper cellular repair and regeneration. Track the number of hours you sleep each night and note any changes in how refreshed you feel in the morning after incorporating sleep-supporting supplements or lifestyle changes.

5. Symptom Monitoring

For those dealing with specific symptoms—such as chronic pain, inflammation, or digestive issues—it's helpful to track these on a daily or weekly basis. Rate the severity of symptoms on a scale from 1–10, and observe any improvements as you implement dietary changes, supplements, or therapies. For example, if reducing joint pain is a goal, track your pain levels before and after introducing an anti-inflammatory diet and PEMF therapy.

Creating a personalized cellular wellness plan is a sustainable way to take control of your health, optimize energy production, and promote long-term vitality. By addressing the foundational pillars of cellular health—nutrition, lifestyle, supplements, and therapies—you can support your body's natural healing processes and reduce the risk of chronic disease. As Benjamin Franklin wisely said, "An ounce of prevention is worth a pound of cure"—by investing in your cellular health today, you lay the foundation for a healthier, more vibrant future.

With the right tools and strategies for tracking your progress, you'll be able to monitor your improvements over time, making adjustments as needed to stay on track with your goals. A personalized cellular wellness plan empowers you to live a healthier, more energized life, knowing you're giving your body the support it needs to thrive.

Next Steps

In the next chapter, we will outline a 30-day action plan designed to provide you with practical steps and daily practices to enhance your cellular health. This actionable guide will help you implement the strategies discussed in this chapter, supporting you in achieving your health goals. With dedication and consistency, you'll be on your way to improved energy, vitality, and overall well-being.

30-Day Action Plan for Enhancing Cellular Health

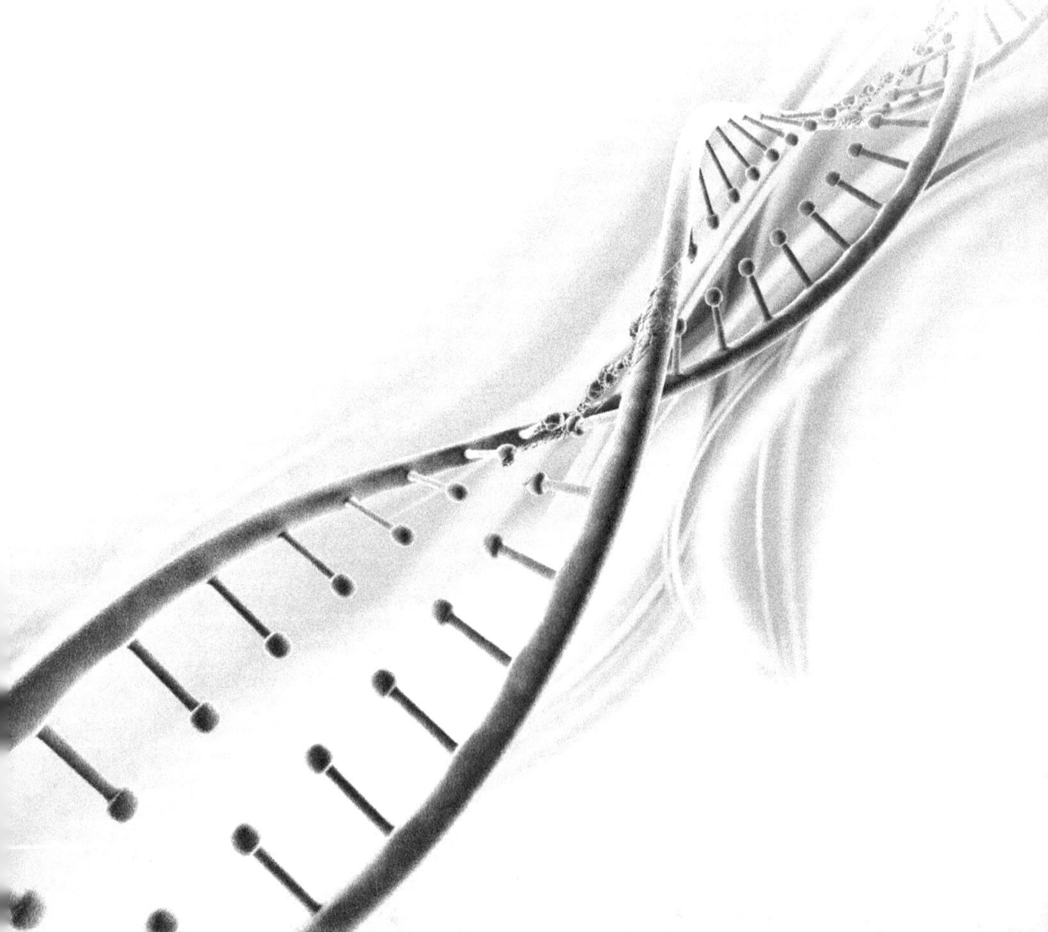

This 30-day action plan outlines daily steps to help you gradually transform your diet and lifestyle, making it easier to integrate these changes sustainably. Each week focuses on building a strong foundation for cellular health, enhancing your habits, and solidifying your new routines. Start slow, increase gradually, monitor progress, and adjust as needed.

Week 1: Foundation Building

Goal: Establish Basic Healthy Habits

- **Day 1:** *Eliminate Processed Foods*
  Start your day with a whole-food breakfast, such as scrambled eggs with fresh fruit. Removing processed foods is essential, as they often contain unhealthy fats, added sugars, and preservatives that can lead to inflammation and oxidative stress at the cellular level.

- **Day 2:** *Add One Serving of Vegetables to Lunch*
  Incorporate a serving of leafy greens or colorful vegetables into your lunch. This increases your intake of antioxidants and essential nutrients vital for cellular repair.

- **Day 3:** *Take a 15–Minute Walk*
  A daily walk enhances circulation and oxygen delivery to your cells, which is crucial for maintaining energy and metabolic function. Aim to drink at least 8 glasses of water today and focus on your breathing to support detoxification.

- **Day 4**: *Introduce a New Fruit to Your Diet*

  Experiment with fruits like berries or kiwi, which are high in antioxidants. Meditate for 5-10 minutes, focusing on your breath to reduce stress, which can negatively impact cellular health.

- **Day 5**: *Plan Meals for the Week*

  Focus on whole foods and include healthy snacks like nuts or Greek yogurt. Meal planning helps prevent impulse eating and supports nutrient-dense choices.

- **Day 6**: *Start Taking a Daily Multivitamin*

  Choose a multivitamin that includes B vitamins and magnesium, both essential for energy production and mitochondrial function.

- **Day 7**: *Reflect on Your Week*

  Journal about your experiences, noting any challenges or successes. Reflection promotes self-awareness and helps adjust future goals.

Week 2: Gradual Enhancements

Goal: Build on Your Foundation with More Intentional Changes

- **Day 8**: *Introduce a New Vegetable at Dinner*

  Try a new vegetable, such as asparagus or beets. Deep breathing exercises for 10 minutes can help enhance your relaxation response.

- **Day 9**: *Meal Prep for the Week Ahead*

  Preparing meals in advance ensures you have healthy options available, reducing the temptation to make unhealthy choices.

- **Day 10**: *Increase Your Walk to 20-30 Minutes*

  Incorporate light stretching and aim to get at least 15 minutes of sunlight exposure, which can boost your vitamin D levels and improve your mood.

- **Day 11**: *Meditate for 10 Minutes*

  Focus on gratitude or positive affirmations to enhance your mental well-being and support cellular repair.

- **Day 12**: *Incorporate Healthy Fats into Your Meals*

  Add sources like avocados and olive oil to your diet, which support brain function and cellular membrane integrity.

- **Day 13**: *Add CoQ10 and Omega-3 Supplements*

  Both supplements support mitochondrial function and reduce inflammation, key factors in cellular health.

- **Day 14**: *Reflect on Your Progress*

  Write down any challenges you faced this week and how you overcame them, fostering a growth mindset.

Week 3: Deepening Practices

Goal: Intensify Your Dietary and Lifestyle Changes

- **Day 15**: *Experiment with a Clean Carnivore or Keto Meal*

  Monitor how your body feels after this dietary change, noting any differences in energy levels or digestion.

- **Day 16**: *Increase Breathing Exercises to 15 Minutes*
  Add visualization techniques to enhance relaxation and focus on energy flow through your body.

- **Day 17**: *Engage in 30–45 Minutes of Varied Exercise*
  Mix cardio and strength training to improve muscle mass and mitochondrial function.

- **Day 18**: *Meditate for 15 Minutes*
  Focus on self-compassion or stress relief techniques, both beneficial for mental and cellular health.

- **Day 19**: *Plan and Prepare Balanced Meals*
  Ensure meals include lean protein and healthy fats to support cellular repair and energy production.

- **Day 20**: *Add Alpha-Lipoic Acid and Acetyl-L-Carnitine to Your Supplement Regimen*
  These supplements can enhance mitochondrial function and support energy metabolism.

- **Day 21**: *Reflect on Your Week*
  Adjust your goals based on what's been working and celebrate your successes.

Week 4: Integrative Lifestyle Changes

Goal: Solidify New Habits and Deepen Your Practice

- **Day 22**: *Prepare Meals for the Upcoming Week*
  Meal prepping helps maintain healthy choices and prevents last-minute unhealthy decisions.

- **Day 23**: *Practice Breathing Exercises for 20 Minutes*
  Use techniques like diaphragmatic breathing and gratitude journaling to promote relaxation and mental clarity.

- **Day 24**: *Engage in 45–60 Minutes of Physical Activity*
  Consider yoga or Pilates to improve flexibility and mindfulness, which can enhance cellular function.

- **Day 25**: *Meditate for 20 Minutes*
  Explore guided sessions that focus on energy and cellular health to deepen your practice.

- **Day 26**: *Focus on Nutrient-Dense Meals*
  Ensure your plate includes a variety of colors, which indicates a range of nutrients to support cellular health.

- **Day 27**: *Introduce Taurine and Glutathione into Your Supplement Routine*
  Both support detoxification and protect against oxidative stress, enhancing cellular health.

- **Day 28**: *Reflect on Your Overall Experience*

  Write about the habits you want to keep moving forward.

Days 29 & 30: Evaluation and Future Planning

- **Day 29**: *Evaluate Your Progress*

  Assess which habits have been beneficial and identify areas for improvement.

- **Day 30**: *Create a Plan for Maintaining Your New Habits*

  Set specific goals for continuing your dietary and holistic practices to ensure lasting changes.

Words of Encouragement for Your 30-Day Cellular Health Journey

Congratulations on taking the first step toward optimizing your self-healing potential and improving your cellular health! Remember, this journey is about progress, not perfection—each day is an opportunity to nourish your body and strengthen its ability to heal itself. You've made a powerful decision to prioritize your well-being, and that's something to be incredibly proud of.

As you move through this 30-day plan, think of it as taking small, meaningful steps toward a much bigger goal. It's not about sprinting toward immediate results; it's about embracing the process and building habits that will support your health in the long run. Healing, especially at the cellular level, takes time, but with consistency, you will begin to feel the transformative effects.

Every time you choose clean, nutrient-dense foods, you are fueling your cells with the energy they need to repair and thrive. Every glass of water you drink helps hydrate and flush your system, supporting detoxification and optimal cellular function. Integrating deep breathing, sunlight, meditation, and gratitude into your daily routine may seem like small actions, but they have profound effects on reducing stress, balancing your nervous system, and boosting your immune response. These simple habits create an environment where your body can focus on healing from the inside out.

Set SMART goals—goals that are Specific, Measurable, Achievable, Realistic, and Timely. Focus on one thing each day, whether it's getting 10 minutes of sunlight, meditating for 5 minutes, or ensuring proper hydration. Each small success adds up. This journey isn't about perfection—it's about long-term, sustainable health. It's okay to have setbacks. Remember, you're not starting over, you're simply continuing your journey. This is a marathon, not a sprint. The real win is building a healthier future for yourself, one step at a time.

"Fix the cells to get and stay well"—this has been my mantra since 1993. By supporting your body's natural healing mechanisms, you're setting yourself up for greater energy, vitality, and resilience. Trust in the process, be kind to yourself, and know that every choice you make toward wellness is an investment in your health for years to come. You've got this! Here's to a healthier, stronger, and more vibrant you. Keep going—you are already making a difference!

The Last Word

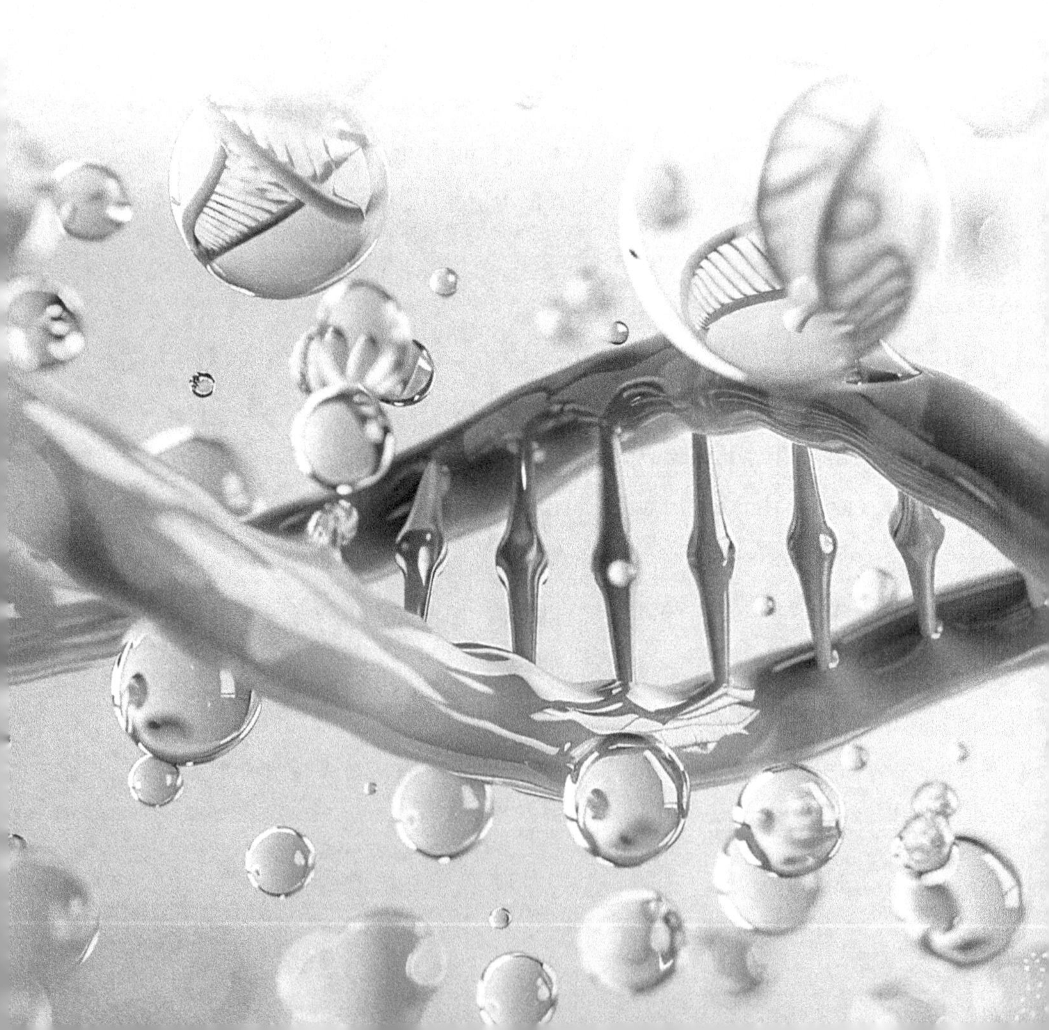

As we reach the conclusion of this transformative journey into cellular health, it becomes clear that the pursuit of well-being is more than just a quest for a healthier body—it's a commitment to understanding the very essence of our biology. Every function in our body, from energy production to cognitive performance, begins at the cellular level. When our cells are healthy, our organs, systems, and entire body thrive. Conversely, when cellular dysfunction occurs, the foundation of health weakens, leaving us vulnerable to disease, fatigue, and premature aging.

"The greatest wealth is health." —Virgil

The good news is that we have incredible control over our cellular health. As we've explored throughout this book, there are numerous strategies, tools, and therapies available to optimize cellular function, repair damage, and prevent future dysfunction. Through nutrition, lifestyle changes, supplementation, and innovative therapies like Bioenergetics, Pulsed Electromagnetic Field (PEMF) therapy, ozone therapy, and IV nutrition—along with mindfulness practices—we can maintain our cells' integrity, enhance their resilience, promote regeneration, and ultimately extend our vitality for years to come.

A central theme of this exploration is the interconnectedness of various factors that influence cellular function. While it may be tempting to focus solely on one area—such as diet or exercise—true cellular health requires a holistic approach. Each aspect of health impacts the others in a way that either supports or undermines cellular function. Consider how these different elements work together to create the foundation for optimal cellular health.

The food we consume provides the building blocks for every process in the body. Nutrients like vitamins, minerals, antioxidants, and amino acids are essential for cell repair and regeneration, energy production, and protection against oxidative stress. A nutrient-dense, anti-inflammatory diet rich in whole foods is foundational to cellular health. Yet, nutrition alone cannot sustain cellular function if sleep, stress management, and exercise are neglected.

"In the middle of difficulty lies opportunity." —Albert Einstein

Stress is one of the most significant contributors to cellular damage. Chronic stress elevates cortisol levels, which, over time, lead to increased inflammation, oxidative damage, and impaired cellular repair. Sleep, too, plays a critical role in cellular regeneration, as most tissue repair and detoxification processes occur during deep sleep. Practicing mindfulness, meditation, and other stress-reduction techniques allows the body to recover from the harmful effects of stress and supports the restoration of cellular balance.

Physical activity is essential for stimulating cellular repair, promoting mitochondrial biogenesis, and improving circulation. Movement helps deliver oxygen and nutrients to cells while removing waste products. Exercise is known to reduce inflammation, improve cardiovascular health, and enhance cognitive function—all of which directly impact cellular health. High-Intensity Interval Training (HIIT) and other forms of exercise significantly improve mitochondrial function, while even gentle activities like walking and yoga contribute to cellular resilience.

Many of these recommendations, such as breathing techniques, grounding, exposure to sunlight, proper hydration, and practicing gratitude and mindfulness, come at little to no cost. Breathing deeply for just a few minutes each day can dramatically reduce stress levels and improve oxygen flow to your cells. Grounding, or connecting with the Earth's energy, can enhance your overall well-being and improve cellular function. Simply soaking in the sun for 15 minutes daily can bolster your vitamin D levels, a vital nutrient for immune support and cellular health, while staying hydrated promotes optimal cellular function and detoxification.

While a healthy diet can provide many of the nutrients our cells need, certain supplements offer targeted support that can fill nutritional gaps, boost energy production, and protect against oxidative stress. Supplements like CoQ10, taurine, phosphatidylcholine, and glutathione provide essential support for mitochondrial health, cellular detoxification, and tissue repair. However, it's important to remember that supplements are most effective when combined with a healthy diet and lifestyle.

For individuals dealing with chronic health conditions, recovering from illness, or looking to optimize performance, innovative therapies like Bioenergetics, PEMF therapy, ozone therapy, and IV nutrition offer additional tools for promoting cellular repair and enhancing energy production. Bioenergetics, which focuses on restoring the body's energetic balance, plays a crucial role in optimizing cellular function. These therapies target specific cellular pathways, reduce inflammation, and improve oxygenation, but are most effective when integrated into a comprehensive wellness plan. One of the most empowering takeaways from this journey is the realization that cellular health is largely within our control. While aging and environmental stressors will inevitably affect our cells over time, the choices we make every day—what we eat, how we move, and how we manage stress—profoundly impact how well our cells function and how resilient they are to damage. A proactive approach to cellular health means taking steps now to prevent future dysfunction. Rather than waiting until disease or fatigue sets in, a cellular wellness plan can help you maintain energy levels, protect against chronic illness, and promote longevity. This proactive mindset encourages us to view health not as a reactive process (responding to symptoms or illness) but as a lifelong commitment to nourishing and supporting our body's most fundamental processes.

The strategies outlined in this book are not meant to be temporary fixes or short-term interventions. Instead, they serve as a foundation for lifelong wellness. Integrating these principles into your daily life is key to sustaining the benefits of cellular health. Long-term improvements come from consistent, sustainable changes. Make small, incremental adjustments to your diet, exercise routine, and lifestyle habits, and stick with them. Over time, these small changes will accumulate into significant improvements in your overall health. Life is dynamic, and so is your health. Be willing to adjust your wellness plan as your needs change. If certain strategies are no longer effective, remain open to exploring new approaches. As you age or experience changes in health, revisit your wellness plan to ensure it still aligns with your goals. Monitoring your progress allows you to see the impact of your efforts and make informed adjustments. Whether you use health tracking apps, journaling, or regular blood tests, tracking improvements in energy levels, sleep, mood, and physical performance can help you stay motivated and identify areas for further optimization.

Staying attuned to your body's signals is essential for maintaining balance. Pay attention to how your body responds to different foods, exercises, supplements, and therapies. Cultivating mindfulness can help you recognize when something is off and encourage you to make necessary changes before cellular dysfunction becomes a more significant issue. It's important to approach your wellness journey with self-compassion and flexibility. There will be days when you don't stick perfectly to your plan, and that's okay. Cellular health is a long-term commitment, and occasional deviations won't derail your progress. Be kind to yourself and focus on getting back on track rather than striving for perfection. The pursuit of cellular wellness isn't just about improving how we feel today; it's also about laying the foundation for long-term health and longevity. As science continues to uncover the mechanisms that contribute to aging, it's becoming increasingly clear that maintaining healthy cellular function is one of the most effective ways to slow the aging process and extend both lifespan and healthspan (the number of years we spend in good health).

"What we think, we become." —Buddha

By focusing on cellular health, we can delay the onset of age-related diseases, improve cognitive function, maintain physical vitality, and enjoy a higher quality of life as we age. This doesn't mean that aging will stop entirely—after all, aging is a natural part of life—but it does mean that we can age with greater resilience, vitality, and independence. As you continue on your wellness journey, remember that your body is a remarkable, self-healing system. Given the right tools and support, your cells have the capacity to repair, regenerate, and maintain balance even in the face of stress and aging. By committing to a cellular wellness plan that focuses on prevention, optimization, and personalization, you are giving your body the best possible chance to thrive.

"Your health is an investment, not an expense." —Unknown

Cellular wellness is not a destination but an ongoing process—a lifelong commitment to nurturing and supporting the very foundation of your health. Whether your goal is to improve energy levels, recover from illness, or simply enjoy a longer, healthier life, the strategies outlined in this book provide a roadmap for empowering yourself with the knowledge and tools you need to take control of your health. As you continue to prioritize your cellular wellness, may you experience the profound benefits of vitality, resilience, and well-being that come from nourishing your body at the deepest level. Fixing the cells to get and stay well is the path to true cellular vitality!

In Gratitude and Healing,
-- Dr. Kelly Brink
www.DrKellyBrink.com

References

1. Abadjian, M. C., Kearns, C., & Cordone, A. J. (2018). Mitochondrial dysfunction and energy metabolism in human aging. *Ageing Research Reviews, 50,* 1-12.

2. Akbari, M., & Kroemer, G. (2019). Mitochondria: The ultimate source of reactive oxygen species (ROS) in aging. *Nature Reviews Molecular Cell Biology, 20*(3), 243-258.

3. Ames, B. N. (2018). Prolonging healthy aging by slowing down the mitochondrial decay of aging. *Annals of the New York Academy of Sciences, 854*(1), 124-148.

4. Baker, M. A., & DeStefano, T. J. (2020). The impact of meditation on stress and cellular aging: A systematic review. *Journal of Integrative Medicine, 18*(1), 30-40.

5. Barja, G. (2019). Towards a unified theory of aging: Mitochondrial decline and free radical damage. *Experimental Gerontology, 119,* 1-8.

6. Benzi, G., & Moretti, A. (2018). Aging and the mitochondrial respiratory chain: Functionality and possible neuroprotective intervention. *Biogerontology, 10*(6), 579-593.

7. Black, D. S., et al. (2015). Mindfulness meditation and reduced inflammation: A randomized controlled trial. *Brain, Behavior, and Immunity, 60,* 80-87.

8. Burkle, A. (2018). DNA repair and PARP in aging. *Journal of Aging and Health, 30*(3), 327-338.

9. Chang, M. (2019). *Mitochondrial Dysfunction: A Functional Medicine Approach to Diagnosis and Treatment.* Self-published.

10. Corder, R. (2019). Polyphenols and cardiovascular health: How we know and what we need to know. *Current Opinion in Lipidology, 30*(3), 240-247.

11. Cresswell, K. M., et al. (2016). Mindfulness and heart rate variability: A study of long-term practitioners. *Applied Psychophysiology and Biofeedback, 41*(1), 1-8.

12. Cutler, R. G., & Mattson, M. P. (2020). Oxidative stress and aging: The role of mitochondrial DNA damage and dysfunction. *Aging Cell, 5*(3), 173-182.

13. DiNicolantonio, J. J., & O'Keefe, J. H. (2018). Nutritional strategies for healthy aging: Coenzyme Q10 and other essential supplements. *Progress in Cardiovascular Diseases, 61*(4), 404-411.

14. El-Haggar, S. M., & Mehanna, N. (2020). The effect of omega-3 fatty acids on mitochondrial function: A systematic review. *Nutrients, 12*(8), 2348.

15. Epel, E. S., et al. (2004). Meditation and telomeres: A study on aging and cellular health. *Psychoneuroendocrinology, 29*(6), 1125-1132.

16. Falkenberg, M., & Larsson, N. G. (2018). Mitochondrial DNA replication and aging: A new connection. *Nature Reviews Genetics, 19*(11), 716-727.

17. Finkel, T., & Holbrook, N. J. (2019). Oxidants, oxidative stress, and the biology of aging. *Nature, 408*(6809), 239-247.

18. Fontana, L., & Partridge, L. (2020). Promoting health and longevity through diet: From model organisms to humans. *Cell, 161*(1), 106-118.

19. Fredrickson, B. L., et al. (2000). The effects of positive emotions on health: The role of gratitude. *Emotion, 2*(2), 134-149.

20. Gladyshev, V. N. (2020). The free radical theory of aging is dead. Long live the damage theory! *Antioxidants & Redox Signaling, 23*(3), 187-200.

21. Harman, D. (2019). The free radical theory of aging. *Journal of Gerontology, 11*(3), 298-300.

22. Jha, A. P., et al. (2010). Meditation training and brain activity: A randomized controlled trial. *The Journal of Alternative and Complementary Medicine, 16*(8), 855-861.

23. Kawamura, N., & Takano, R. (2020). Exercise-induced mitochondrial biogenesis and its relationship to aging. *Aging and Disease, 11*(3), 453-468.

24. Kheirbek, M. A., & Sahay, A. (2020). Mindfulness, meditation, and cognitive resilience: Evidence from neurobiological studies. *Trends in Cognitive Sciences, 24*(1), 15-22.

25. Kirtman, B. P., et al. (2018). Cortisol levels and the stress response: The role of meditation. *Biological Psychiatry, 83*(5), 474-481.

26. Klein, R. F., & Simmons, S. B. (2019). Taurine and brain health: Neuroprotection and cellular repair mechanisms. *Neurochemical Research, 44*(2), 256-266.

27. Know, L. (2018). *Mitochondria and the Future of Medicine: The Key to Understanding Disease, Chronic Illness, Aging, and Life Itself.* Chelsea Green Publishing.

28. Lanza, I. R., & Nair, K. S. (2020). Mitochondrial metabolism: Implications for exercise and aging. *Journal of Physiology, 587*(23), 5593-5607.

29. Li, J., & Xu, P. (2018). Ozone therapy in inflammation, immune response, and cellular detoxification. *Journal of Inflammation Research, 11*, 527-539.

30. Liu, J., & Ames, B. N. (2019). Reducing mitochondrial decay with age through mitochondrial nutrients. *Annals of the New York Academy of Sciences, 1031*(1), 508-510.

31. Luong, C. C., & Shanley, P. S. (2020). Sleep and cellular repair: A new understanding of sleep's impact on aging. *Cell Metabolism, 22*(3), 611-621.

32. Mahoney, C. R., & Felson, M. P. (2020). Methylene blue as a neuroprotective agent: Cellular mechanisms and clinical applications. *Neurotherapeutics, 17*(1), 1-11.

33. Massey, H. (2019). *Energy 4 Life: How to Charge Your Body Battery and Optimize Your Control System.* NES Health.

34. Mattson, M. P. (2019). Exercise enhances mitochondrial biogenesis and neuroplasticity: Implications for brain health and aging. *Current Opinion in Clinical Nutrition and Metabolic Care, 13*(6), 536-541.

35. Merry, T. L., & Ristow, M. (2020). Mitohormesis and exercise: Hormetic effects on mitochondrial function and aging. *Exercise and Sport Sciences Reviews, 46*(3), 180-187.

36. Mozaffarian, D. (2020). Omega-3 fatty acids and health: Broad benefits, balanced risks. *Journal of the American College of Cardiology, 58*(20), 2047-2060.

37. Myers, M. R., & Porges, S. W. (2021). Polyvagal theory and its application in understanding mindfulness and meditation's effects on cellular stress. *Psychosomatic Medicine, 83*(1), 46-54.

38. Noda, K., & Koike, S. (2020). PEMF therapy for chronic pain and inflammation: Evidence from clinical studies. *Pain Medicine, 21*(5), 1184-1193.

39. Packer, L., & Cadenas, E. (2019). The role of antioxidants in cellular defense and aging: A comprehensive review. *Free Radical Biology and Medicine, 50*(8), 915-921.

40. Pal, G. K., & Nanda, N. (2019). Oxidative stress and mitochondrial dysfunction in aging: Therapeutic interventions and exercise adaptations. *Journal of Clinical and Diagnostic Research, 13*(4), LE01-LE06.

41. Passos, J. F., & von Zglinicki, T. (2019). Senescent cells and the accumulation of DNA damage with age. *Trends in Molecular Medicine, 15*(9), 429-436.

42. Peng, C., & Sies, H. (2019). Vitamin E and cellular health: Molecular mechanisms and clinical relevance. *Nutrients, 11*(9), 2059.

43. Powers, S. K., & Jackson, M. J. (2020). Exercise-induced oxidative stress: Cellular mechanisms and impact on muscle function. *Physiological Reviews, 88*(4), 1243-1276.

44. Redman, L. M., &Ravussin, E. (2020). Caloric restriction and mitochondrial function: Impact on longevity and aging. *Nature Reviews Endocrinology, 17*(1), 61-72.

45. Rehman, J., & Weisel, R. D. (2018). Stem cells and regenerative medicine: Cellular mechanisms and clinical applications. *The Lancet, 379*(9820), 1759-1767.

46. Richardson, A. G., & Hausman, S. (2020). The role of cellular detoxification in aging and longevity. *Current Opinion in Toxicology, 16*(3), 1-6.

47. Ristow, M., & Schmeisser, S. (2019). Mitochondrial hormesis and its role in longevity regulation. *Molecular Cell, 21*(6), 190-203.

48. Rosenberg, M. (2004). The effect of mindfulness on cellular aging: Telomere length. *The Journal of Psychoneuroendocrinology, 29*(6), 712-719.

49. Schieber, M., & Chandel, N. S. (2020). ROS function in redox signaling and oxidative stress. *Current Biology, 24*(10), R453-R462.

50. Schulz, T. J., & Spiegelman, B. M. (2019). Cellular energy sensing and metabolism: Mitochondrial biogenesis and beyond. *Trends in Endocrinology & Metabolism, 18*(4), 228-235.

51. Shallenberger, F. (2011). *Principles and Applications of Ozone Therapy: A Practical Guideline for Physicians.* Self-published.

52. Silva, S. D., & Trindade, E. P. (2019). The impact of taurine supplementation on mitochondrial function: A meta-analysis. *Mitochondrion, 47*, 162-168.

53. Smith, R. A., & Murphy, M. P. (2019). Antioxidants and mitochondrial health: Cellular targets and clinical applications. *Trends in Pharmacological Sciences, 31*(11), 605-612.

54. Sullivan, C. S., & Horwitz, R. I. (2020). Meditation, prayer, and their effect on cellular aging and health outcomes: A review. *Mind–Body Medicine, 15*(1), 22-36.

55. Tanaka, T., & Manini, T. M. (2020). Mitochondrial decline and its role in cellular aging. *Journal of Aging Research, 45*(4), 353-362.

56. Wallace, D. C., & Fan, W. (2020). The role of mitochondrial DNA in cellular aging and disease. *Nature Reviews Genetics, 13*(12), 712-725.

57. Whitten, A. (2018). *Red Light Therapy.* Energy Blueprint.

58. Wood, A. M., et al. (2010). Gratitude and health: The role of positive emotion in stress and immune function. *Personality and Individual Differences, 49*(8), 930-935.